6/13/11
$19.95
Amzn

Withdra

SATURDAY IS FOR FUNERALS

SATURDAY IS FOR FUNERALS

Unity Dow & Max Essex

HARVARD UNIVERSITY PRESS

Cambridge, Massachusetts, and London, England

2010

Printed in the United States of America

Library of Congress Cataloging-in-Publication Data

Dow, Unity.
Saturday is for funerals / Unity Dow and Max Essex.
p. ; cm.
Includes bibliographical references and index.
ISBN 978-0-674-05077-8 (alk. paper)
I. AIDS (Disease)—Botswana.   I. Essex, Myron.   II. Title.
[DNLM: 1. Acquired Immunodeficiency Syndrome—epidemiology—
Botswana.   2. Acquired Immunodeficiency Syndrome—epidemiology—HIV
Infections. WC 503.4 HB4 D744s 2010]
RA643.86.B55D69 2010
614.5'993920096883—dc22   2009052264

This book is
dedicated to our children,
Cheshe, Tumisang, Natasha,
Holly, and Carrie

Contents

Preface

HIV infections have already killed tens of millions of people, most of them in Africa. Southern Africa has been hit hardest. Botswana, the setting for this book, is in the middle of southern Africa, the "hot zone" for HIV/AIDS.

It has been said that many more are affected by AIDS than just those who are infected with HIV: orphans have lost parents, parents have lost children, spouses have lost partners, schools have lost teachers, farms have lost farmers. So behind every HIV infection is some form of personal tragedy for others—not just for the deceased, the sick person, or the stigmatized individual who is infected. *Saturday Is for Funerals* is designed to reveal these real-life tragedies, and to build on them to help explain this unprecedented epidemic of death and destruction.

HIV is a stealth type of killer. It sneaks in through events of human bonding: conjugation and childbirth. Events that should be sacred and wonderful, not the seeds of death. The virus usually stays hidden in the body for a few years, gradually rising to strangle the immune system—the ultimate death sentence.

The epidemic of HIV/AIDS has often been described as a calamity that could destroy Africa. In the year 2000, the World Health Organization estimated that 85 percent of fifteen-year-olds in Botswana would eventually die of AIDS; life expectancy would fall by forty-four years, from a previously projected seventy-three years to just twenty-nine. This could have happened, but it won't. It won't happen because of action by political leaders and community leaders, nurses and doctors, research scientists, and educators of all types. New techniques are now available that dramatically reduce rates of transmission by mothers to their children. New therapies can save the lives of most people with AIDS. We have gained intricate knowledge about HIV and how it spreads. But we still have no vaccine, inadequate financial resources, and a relative lack of physicians and nurses. Too often there is also a lack of political will. When taken together, these limitations are usually devastating. This is what happened in Africa.

While this book is not a road map for success, it should help the reader appreciate how individuals and a country responded at a time of crisis. As authors, we come from different backgrounds. Unity comes from a background of law, ethics, and human rights; Max, from a background of academia and medical research. Unity is a native of Botswana who has lived through the experiences of the AIDS epidemic reflected in this book. Max has been involved in AIDS research from the earliest days of the U.S. epidemic in 1982, and in Botswana since 1996.

As the conduct of prevention, treatment, and research began to interfere with issues of confidentiality, distributive justice, and human rights, we realized that our experiences were complementary—perhaps even synergistic if combined to tell the story of AIDS in Africa. In the chapters that follow, Unity recounts the personal, human experiences of the epidemic among the people of Botswana. Max presents scientific and medical explanations that apply not only to the individual stories told but also to the global fight against HIV/AIDS. We believe that the experiences of Botswana provide numerous lessons that the world needs to learn.

Our special thanks to Esmond Harmsworth for advice about publication; Michael Fisher, Julie Hagen, and Anne Zarella for preparation and editing; and Barry Bloom, Cheshe Dow, Elizabeth Essex, Doug Given, Lendsey Melton, Karl Stahl, Barbara Wu, and Soon-Young Yoon for constructive criticism. No Motswana can read an HIV/AIDS story without recognizing himself or herself in bits of the narrative, and no one should read an HIV/AIDS story without recognizing that it holds a larger story beyond the literal words used in the text. The characters whose stories are told in this book provided us with material necessary not just to tell their stories, but also to inform readers about the collective experience of the epidemic of AIDS in Africa. We thank them, and we hope that they will find that we have treated their tragedies, hopes, and joys with respect. This book gives them an opportunity to be heard as well as a mechanism to help educate others. It is our hope that the world will respond to their voices in many positive ways.

SATURDAY IS FOR FUNERALS

Introduction

IN NOVEMBER 1996, a close member of Unity's family, a cousin, died after "a long illness." It seems likely that she was infected with HIV in August 1988. At that time, she was attacked by a ferocious flulike syndrome that pinned her to her bed for at least five days. She recovered from the flu, but her body seemed to be fighting an invisible demon. At first it seemed she had won the fight. In retrospect, she probably had not. The monster had been deceitful and had merely raised the white flag to lull her into a false sense of security. About six years later it reared its head again; no pretenses, no hiding. Over a two-year period, the cousin's flesh seemed to melt away from between the skin and the bones. No sores, no diarrhea— just a melting away, so that by the time she died, the skin clung to her bones so tightly that it seemed it would break during her baths.

Then another cousin died; then another, then a friend, then an aunt, then a coworker . . .

From the midnineties until about two years ago, death and funerals in Botswana were so common that you could not plan any other event for Saturday mornings. As if that were not enough, funerals started claiming weekdays as well. Bodies were piling up in mortuaries; cemeteries were crowded on Saturdays; the dead had to be buried so the ill could be tended to.

Things were getting out of hand. Even cultural practices had to be changed. While grave digging had always been a midnight task, now young men could be seen on late afternoons digging graves for friends and relatives. The traditional year-long mourning period for widows and widowers had to be shortened, for who would tend the sick and bury the dead in the meantime? Hospitals were spilling over and family members had to help.

As the AIDS epidemic expanded, modern medicine was failing, admitting publicly to being unable to restore the health of those infected. So people looked elsewhere, to healing churches and traditional doctors. Diviners and healers, and a new breed that was a bit of both, sprang up everywhere. Bones were cast and blame was assigned to enemies real and imagined. From the start, AIDS has been a disease made for myths and witchcraft. The following fictional account of a divination is based on a session that Unity attended:

> "I see a thin woman entering your home as if she belongs there, yet perhaps she does not quite belong. She must be a relative or perhaps a friend?" the diviner asks as he concentrates on his bones, a frown of concern evident, as he seems to try to puzzle out some meaning from the bones.
>
> Before Mara can answer, the bone thrower shakes his head, clearly in deep thought, concerned at what his bones are telling him. He looks up and commands Mara, "Pick them up and breathe life into them."
>
> Mara collects the eight or so small pieces of bone, and, cupping them in her hands, blows into them.
>
> "Say after me, 'I ask you once more.'"
>
> "I ask you once more," chants Mara.
>
> "Tell me what troubles me."

"Tell me what troubles me," she repeats after the diviner.

"What is eating me and my family?"

"What is eating me and my family?"

"Who is scattering us?"

"Who is scattering us?"

"Who is killing us?"

"Who is killing us?"

"Now throw them," orders the diviner.

Mara throws the bones, and they scatter in a pattern she cannot possibly understand, but she has all the confidence that the diviner can. One particular piece, which looks more like a piece of hard plastic or perhaps ivory, rather than bone, with intricate engravings, jumps from the rest and falls with its sharper point pointing west. It seemed to leap from the rest with a life of its own. Mara draws in a sharp breath. Although she cannot interpret the fall, she is shaken by this, since she understands that west, the direction of sunset, is also the direction of darkness and death. The direction of the end. The direction of hopelessness. Of nothingness. She stifles a scream that is threatening to escape from her and at once constricting her throat. The diviner looks up sharply but says nothing.*

If we choose to despair, we can find support for our hopelessness in questions that arise on both the personal and the policy level. What are young adults keen on starting a family to do, when procreation might mean infection? What is a young mother to do when faced with the choice between breastfeeding and formula feeding, when both have their dangers? When queues for treatment are long,

* Unity Dow, *Far and Beyon'*, 2nd ed. (San Francisco: Aunt Lute Books, 2002), 3–4.

who should be at the head of the line? Are some lives more valuable than others? Should routine testing be promoted? Who benefits? Who gets hurt? Where should the balance be struck? These are moral and ethical questions, and they are endless.

This book presents true stories of people's lives, as well as the scientific explanations behind the events. Only the names have been changed. In the final analysis, understanding how people live and love is the key to understanding how and whether the scientific breakthroughs will work, and how to redesign them so they will work better.

A Family of Funerals

The Epidemic

MY PARENTS ARE IN THEIR SEVENTIES and this makes them the senior members of their respective extended families. Hardly a wedding or a funeral in the neighborhood or the family can take place without their attendance. My mother says the good thing about weddings is that they can be planned. Funerals usually cannot, as you cannot be sure when death will strike, but with the climbing rate of AIDS deaths, funerals are taking up every Saturday, squeezing weddings out of the agenda altogether. Nature has gone crazy, she says. There had always been a balance between death and birth, but not anymore.

"We are burying babies with their parents! How can there be a future?"

It is a Saturday in 2007 and my mother has not been to a funeral in two weeks; she is grateful for the respite. She whips out three funeral programs. "Here. You may not have heard about these deaths. She was my . . ." She explains how she was related to the three deceased persons. One was related to her through her great-great-grandmother and the other in some equally distant way. She does not think their relationship was so distant, and she rebukes me for not taking blood relations seriously.

She keeps funeral programs, like many other people, because so many people are dying that it is difficult to keep up.

"If you have not seen someone for a while and you meet their mother, you are afraid to ask after them. Perhaps they have died and you have not heard. It was never like this before. You must remember people's children and be sure to ask how they are. How can you ask about people who may be dead?"

I remind her that things have improved; she has not been to a funeral in two full weeks! My youngest brother, who lives at home with my parents, pipes up that he has not dug a grave in three weeks. He, too, is grateful for the break. He cannot remember a Friday night in 2004 and 2005 that he did not dig a grave, nor a week during those years when he did not have to ride a truck to collect firewood for one funeral or another.

For my mother, the funeral of a relative or a neighbor—and in a village setting, these terms are defined very liberally—demands attendance at evening prayers from the time of the person's death to the date of the funeral, which would typically be the next Saturday at 6:00 AM, as well as an overnight vigil the night before the funeral. In the case of particularly close relatives, she must spend nights at the home of the deceased with other senior members of the family. My mother is generally dissatisfied by the funeral attendance of most of her children; she feels we do not attend enough funerals.

"Who is going to bury me, when I am dead, if my children do not bury others?"

My sister jokes that we are big enough as a family to bury our own. My mother fails to appreciate the humor. "I am going to be eaten by dogs, the way you all carry on! My funeral will be the talk of the village!" She exaggerates, but she is correct. Since AIDS started claiming lives with such regularity that some families have had to quickly bury one family member during the week to make way for another over the weekend, we have not been able to keep up with funeral demands. A typical sanction for punishing a family whose members do not attend the funerals of others is for the crowd to attend a funeral in that family but not to eat the food provided. It is considered the height of insult to be left with pots of food and no one to share them with, and my mother lives in fear of this ultimate shame. My brother tries to mollify her: "But I attend funerals. I dig graves all the time! You should not worry."

"Yes, at least dogs will not eat my feet. But will anyone eat with you, afterwards? Your brothers never attend funerals."

Funerals are exhausting undertakings. For the closest female neighbors and relatives, during the days leading to the funeral they have to brew tea, bake *diphaphatha* bread, cook sorghum porridge with spinach or cabbage and, perhaps, goat meat or beef. For the close male relatives and neighbors, the work involved during the days before a funeral includes collecting firewood and killing, skinning, and preparing a goat or cow, if the family can afford such a luxury. The night before the funeral is particularly busy. Men dig the grave and cook the meat; women cook the sorghum porridge, maize porridge, and samp that must be served at every funeral, while brewing tea for everyone throughout an overnight vigil of singing and preaching.

By 6:00 AM the food is ready and the funeral proper begins. This typically involves preaching, hymn singing, prayers, speeches, reading of messages written by family and friends to the departed, and finally interment at the grave. By 11:00 AM the food is served, and by the afternoon women are washing plates and utensils and men are returning borrowed chairs, tables, and big cooking pots. The following day, Sunday, close family members assemble to wash the deceased's clothes and pack them away until they can be distributed at a special family gathering convened for that purpose.

Death therefore takes up more than just the Saturday for the funeral, and when I asked my mother how many funerals she had been to during 2004, the year she considers to have been the worst, she gave the following account:

"I can't remember all of them, they have been many. But let me see . . . Let me count only those related to me, otherwise we will never finish.

"First there was your uncle Rra Tekanyo. He was always an unfaithful man, torturing my sister with his behavior. Always running around with women, young and old, but when he fell sick, we did not even suspect the plague. It was before we knew a lot about this disease. And he passed it on to my sister. She too later died. It was such an embarrassment at their age to die of a young person's disease. He really exposed my sister to ridicule. Of course it was hush-hush.

"Then it was Thabiso, the child of my sister. [For my mother's generation, the terms "niece" and "cousin" hardly exist. They have sisters, brothers, parents and children, uncles and aunts.] Such a beautiful young girl, I don't want to remember how she suffered. She left a child, three years old at the time, and she was adopted by Thabiso's sister. I remember there was a family fight when someone said she died of AIDS, and the family raked her over the coals for that. It was quite a scandal when she said she heard it from Thabiso's own sister.

"Then came Nnana, child of my brother. She too was sick for a long time. She left two children and one of them, the younger one, died a year later. He too died of the same thing. That poor child! The diarrhea and mouth sores! It was sad to watch.

"But remember that Nnana's own brother died, too. I know it was TB but I cannot say that it was this disease. Maybe it was. But he drank a lot and did not eat well. How can we be sure that it was not something else? He left a wife and lots of children. At least the children were not so young; some were in high school already.

"Then there was Mma Monica, your favorite. That was a sad one. I don't want to dwell on that one too much. Her own mother, my sister, died of childbirth when I was only ten or fifteen years old but I can still hear her wails, and then she too had to die such a sad painful death. No, I don't want to talk about her.

"Let me see . . . after Mma Monica comes Monica herself. Of course she did not die but she nearly did. She suffered before going on ARVs, and she had cancer. Cervical cancer, the doctors said. Let's hope all is well. She looks well anyway. She has gained a lot of weight, but the treatment! *Joo!* If anyone was saved by humor, it was that woman. She could laugh and cry and make you laugh and cry with her. She suffered, my child, she suffered!

"Closer to home here, Lekang died, child of my sister, a sister with whom we shared a breast. ["A sister with whom we shared a breast" is a sibling, as opposed to a cousin.] She was a naughty woman, I must admit. As a young woman, and even later when she was married, she never stopped with her naughtiness. Couldn't keep to one man! The consequences of running around with many partners are harsh, I must say. Harsh! She left five children. With her gone, only one of the children stayed in school for any length of time. Two of the girls now have children. One lost one child to AIDS and promptly replaced him with another. Pure madness, how AIDS is killing children! When you see a pregnant girl, you wonder, is she carrying death or a child?

"And my other sister, also a sister with whom I shared a breast, her grandchild died. I remember she became confused, saying strange things, running around like a mad person. And then she went into a coma and died. Her husband was sick first. There was a lot of finger pointing, but how does that help? When a dog is dead, it is dead! But now he is on ARVs. He is raising their two young children and they seem to be doing well.

"I can't name them all. They are many. For example, my brother Rra Thato—my grandmother and his grandmother were closely related—he lost two children within two months. Both girls, and both left young children. Only God knows where the children's fathers are. My brother later died. I think it was from a painful heart.

"And I remember that your cousin Tshepi came with her ailing husband to Thato's funeral; he could hardly speak. A month later he too was dead! Now Tshepi is ill; she claims to have all kinds of conditions with fancy unpronounceable names but the truth is that she has AIDS! How could she have escaped? They were trying to have children for years without success; of course she was exposed to the virus.

"But now things are much better. During those years, you had ten to twelve funerals at the same time. That group trying to sing and that one too. I can easily count fifty funerals I attended in one year. Easily! Every Saturday, there was a funeral."

❖

For Botswana, the new century began with an almost unimaginable death toll from AIDS. After initial infection with HIV, it usually takes a person eight to twelve years to die. A few people develop lethal disease within a year or two, and a few survive twenty years after infection, but such cases are rare. When one designs education programs to prevent AIDS, this long and variable incubation period before disease develops causes great confusion. With most infectious diseases, such as influenza, measles, or smallpox, the disease and death, when it occurs, come soon after infection.

A lack of understanding about how and why it takes so long to develop the disease led some to proclaim that HIV wasn't really the cause of AIDS, just a passenger virus that did no harm. A few denialists have claimed that AIDS doesn't even exist as a real disease, or if it does, it is caused by the use of illicit drugs, not the sexually transmitted virus. If this is so, it follows, why use condoms for AIDS prevention? The dissemination of such disinformation by President Mbeki of South Africa and other denialists may have resulted in the loss of many lives in that country. South Africa, with six million HIV infections, has more than any other country.

Botswana is at ground zero, right in the middle of the most severe epidemic of HIV/AIDS in southern Africa. It is commonly stated that the first AIDS case in Botswana was diagnosed in 1984. Though this may be true, that person was probably infected elsewhere, as the epidemic of HIV in the region did not really begin until the late 1980s. At about that time, a decade or so after the epidemic was established in East and Central Africa, the prevalence of HIV infection rose rapidly in Botswana. By 1996 or 1997 new infections, or the incidence of HIV, had rapidly expanded to cause prevalence rates of more than 30 percent in young adults. Because few cases of AIDS disease or death were evident at this time, owing to the long incubation period, people did not appreciate the severity of the epidemic. The sexual transmission of HIV from infected individuals is most efficient when one has been infected recently. A peak in virus production occurs a month or so after the initial infection, when more than 100,000 infectious viruses may be present in a single drop of blood.

For Unity's parents, 2004 and 2005 were the years of constant funerals. This fits well with a peak time period of 1996 for new HIV infections, followed by an eight- to ten-year period for progression to death from the disease. By 2006, antiretroviral drugs (ARVs) to treat AIDS were becoming widely available in Botswana. Although not a cure in the sense of eliminating the HIV virus from the body, the combination of three drugs in the treatment designated HAART (highly active antiretroviral treatment) usually prevents death and restores the AIDS patient to relative health. The drug treatment, if faithfully followed, cuts HIV reproduction rates dramatically but doesn't stop virus production completely. Once begun, adherence to the HAART regimen is essential, as failure to take the pills on schedule results in a rapid activation of the quiescent viruses, whose DNA has now been stored in the patient's chromosomes. Failure to adhere to the schedule for taking HAART drugs sometimes occurs because the medications cause nausea or other side effects. In a few patients, but not many, the side effects of the drugs can seem as bad as the disease itself. The effects are similar in principle to the toxic effects seen in cancer patients on therapy, but generally much less severe.

At the funerals that follow deaths from AIDS, the cause of death is often camouflaged—as pneumonia, perhaps, or severe diarrhea or tuberculosis. Here again, the disease of AIDS lends itself to confusion, denial, and cover-up, because the signs and symptoms are so similar to those seen in a range of other diseases. This is because HIV targets primarily lymphocytes and macrophages. These cells provide the backbone of immunity. As more and more immune cells are killed by HIV replication, the immune system fails. As the immune system fails, opportunistic infections flourish. Some, such as the yeast *Candida albicans,* cause severe thrush in the mouth, esophagus, and other mucous membranes. TB, already present in many people, especially those in developing countries, is usually kept under control by the immune system. When the immune system fails, the *Mycobacterium tuberculosis* bacteria are unchecked and pulmonary or extrapulmonary tuberculosis appears as a severe disease. Nnana had diarrhea and mouth sores. The diarrhea could have been due to bacteria or protozoa that grow better in the gut when the immune system is damaged. The mouth sores could have been caused by yeast, or by a herpesvirus. Herpes can cause systemic disease after

HIV destroys lymphocytes. Bacteria in the gut cause diarrhea, failure to adsorb food nutrients, wasting, and emaciation.

A grandchild of Mma Monica's sister became confused, running around like a mad person before going into a coma and dying. HIV can also infect the brain, causing dementia. As the immune system is destroyed, some opportunistic fungi, such as *Cryptococcus neoformans,* cause infections of the meninges, the membranous cover of the brain. This usually occurs only during late-stage AIDS. Death normally follows soon after the diagnosis.

Obviously you don't have to have HIV/AIDS to get TB, diarrhea, or herpes ulcers. HIV just makes them worse—much worse. This wide range of associated diseases also lends itself to denial concerning the cause of AIDS. Condoms don't prevent TB, but they may prevent death from TB by keeping the body free of HIV. The cause of death is rarely listed as AIDS—it is usually something else.

In Botswana, siblings, parents, or children with AIDS do not seem to be avoided by their families. There seems to be a subconscious acceptance that the AIDS disease can be acquired only by sexual exposure, blood transfusion, dirty needles, or mother-to-infant transmission. The stigma or shame of having HIV/AIDS is presumably limited to the sexual exposure, with its implication of promiscuity or unfaithfulness. Thus it was quite a scandal when Thabiso's sister told some family members that Thabiso had AIDS. And the family seemed to know that Lekang was a "naughty woman." In the Botswana culture, families nurse their diseased children, and willingly accept orphaned children, even knowing or suspecting they are infected with HIV. This is both admirable and appropriate, because HIV poses no danger to uninfected family members, except through sex, childbirth, or breastfeeding.

Rra Tekanyo was an unfaithful older man who "ran around" with younger and older women, and ultimately infected Unity's mother's sister, who also died. In southern Africa, rates of HIV infection rapidly increase among young women age sixteen to twenty-four. In this age range, three or four times as many women may be infected as men. This is because older men frequently have sex with younger women, but younger men rarely have sex with older women. And in Africa, more women are infected than men. Why this is so is not clear, but one possibility may be that HIV is more easily transmitted from infected men to women than from infected women to men. Whatever the reason, the highest infection rates in women coincide with the peak age of childbearing, putting large numbers of infants at risk. Without drug treatment to prevent transmission from the mother, in regions of peak prevalence, up to one in eight infants may be infected with HIV, and many others, even though not infected, become orphans. Because of the variability in time to death after infection, however, one cannot be sure that Rra Tekanyo infected the sister, even though he died first, or whether she infected him.

Monica nearly died before "going on ARVs," which is the same as highly active antiretroviral therapy, or HAART. This was the experience of many after 2004. Although HAART treatment began to be followed in Botswana in 2002, the limited availability of drugs and expertise meant that HAART was not available to all who needed it until 2005 or 2006. In Africa, according to United Nations AIDS (UNAIDS) guidelines, HAART treatment is initiated only when patients have an AIDS-defining illness, such as TB or serious wasting, or when the immune system has lost about 70 to 80 percent of the immune cells. The primary cells needed to orchestrate immunity, the T4 cells, are targeted and directly killed by HIV.

Although HAART treatment is well tolerated by many, especially after the patient learns how to schedule the medications with food intake, it seems that Monica experienced the nausea and other gastrointestinal disturbances that can accompany treatment. Monica also suffered from cancer of the uterine cervix. Although the direct cause of this disease is another virus, human papillomavirus, it is possible that the loss of immunity due to HIV/AIDS could have caused the cervical cancer to develop or progress. This cancer is usually surgically treated by removal of the womb.

Unity's mother also said, "When you see a pregnant girl, you wonder, is she carrying death or a child?" Up to 40 percent of children born to HIV-infected mothers may themselves become infected. Some become infected while in the womb, others during the process of birth, and some while breastfeeding. Transmission from mother to child can be dramatically reduced during all these stages with chemoprophylaxis, which involves some of the same drugs used for HAART therapy. Dramatic progress has been made in this area, and much research is still under way.

The AIDS epidemic in southern Africa arose about a decade later than the epidemic in Central Africa and East Africa, which was evident by the early 1980s. The virus subtype that caused the epidemic in southern Africa, HIV-1C, is different from the viruses that caused earlier epidemics. It is arguable that the HIV-1C may be easier to transmit, as the countries in this region have infection rates three to five times higher than the rates observed in other regions of Africa. All of the eight or ten countries with the highest infection rates in the world are in this region. Some, such as Botswana, South Africa, and Namibia, have the highest rates of personal income in sub-Saharan Africa, but others, such as Malawi, Mozambique, and Zambia, are very poor. At least in southern Africa, national poverty rates are not correlated with rates of HIV infection.

In the early days of the epidemic in Africa, civil unrest and armed conflict were thought by some to be important risk factors for HIV infection. But this certainly could not apply in Botswana, which had been peaceful and well governed for decades before the epidemic began. If societal disruption has played any role in expanding the epidemic in Botswana, it could be through urbanization and the mobility associated with increased affluence. Younger people are more likely to be better educated and more mobile—and more sexually active. And the young skilled workers who move to cities such as Gaborone still maintain strong ties to the villages of their parents. At the early stages of the epidemic, the cities had higher rates of HIV infection. As the epidemic progressed, the smaller villages began to catch up.

The first diagnosis of clinical AIDS was made in America, when homosexual men in several cities were found to have unusual illnesses that were not ordinarily seen in young adults. HIV was identified and characterized a few years later. By 1985 tests were available to screen blood, but HAART drug combinations were not available to save lives through treatment until the mid-1990s. Initially the antiretroviral drugs were very expensive and it was thought that only experienced infectious disease experts should administer them and monitor the patients on treatment. This approach was excessively cautious. By 2002 to 2004, prices of ARVs fell precipitously as generic copies of many drugs were produced in countries such as India and Brazil and made available for widespread distribution. It soon became obvious that HAART treatment worked in Africa just as well as it did in the wealthy countries of the north.

As more and more AIDS patients are successfully treated and kept alive in countries like Botswana, the number of those infected will go up, not down. The total number infected, or the prevalence, stays the same if the rate of new infections is equivalent to the death rate. If death rates are reduced by 70 to 80 percent through effective HAART treatment, the rate of new infections, or the incidence, must decrease by at least the same amount just to stay even.

I Know You Still Love Me

Sexual Transmission

DIVORCES IN BOTSWANA are heard by the High Court; that is how seriously the country views marriage. By the time a marriage occurs, there will have been, at the very minimum, six family meetings, starting with those involving close family and progressing to those involving easily sixty or more extended family members. During the weeks, sometimes months, of family meetings and negotiations, small and big feasts are enjoyed, during which presents of *bogadi* cattle, firewood, and clothes are handed over to the bride's family by the husband's. By the time the couple says their Western-influenced "I do's" before the marriage officer or Catholic priest or minister of religion, and an equally Western-style wedding party is held under white tents, all the customary aspects of the marriage process have been concluded. Parents, uncles, and aunts have given their advice, and the recurring message is simple: "Not two people but two families have just been joined in marriage, and nothing, not even death, is expected to end the relationship." In fact, according to custom a deceased woman can remain married to a living man. So death does not, per se, end marriage under traditional law.

The marriage of Daisy and Kopano would have been no different. At the time of their wedding he was thirty-three and she was only twenty-two; he was a clerk and she was a nurse: two educated people setting out to start a family and promising that they would stick together "in sickness and in health." Twenty-two and without a pre-marital child—a circumstance that was becoming a rarity in Botswana; Daisy's face had been covered in white lace to signify this. There had been such hope!

Ten years on, though, they were in the High Court—in my courtroom—standing across from each other and without the presence of family and friends, having come to end the marriage. It had all started with joyous singing and extravagant feasting. Now it was ending, and in Kopano's voice as he gave evidence in support of his case, there was not the usual acrimony that attends most divorces, but rather a sadness, perhaps even embarrassment.

"My wife has behaved in such a manner that it would be unreasonable to expect me to continue to live with her. My marriage has broken down irretrievably."

The statement sounded rehearsed, as if he were afraid to move from his prepared script, lest he falter. His lawyer urged him to go on, to give examples of the unreasonable behavior he says his wife engaged in. His wife looked up at him from across the room, almost challenging him. She was a beautiful woman and she stood with poise and confidence. She was wearing maroon lipstick and when she pursed her lips, which she had a tendency to do, she seemed to be flirting or about to break into a smile.

The man faltered, grabbed the glass of water in front of him, and raised it to his mouth, only to put it down again without drinking. His hands were trembling. His lawyer was having no better time; she was fumbling with the papers in front of her.

The courtroom was quiet.

Others were waiting to have their turn and no doubt they were imagining themselves up there, publicly admitting that they had been unable to make their marriage work. No doubt many, in filing for divorce, had to go against the wishes of their family. "*Ngwnaka itshoke*"—My child, persevere—would have been the entreaty. That final walk into the High Court in Botswana would have taken immense courage. A few—not many, from the number of people in the gallery—may have brought a friend or relative for support.

What is more, when a marriage fails, it is a walk that is more often than not taken by women, not men. Botswana society will tolerate a man who, estranged from his wife, takes a public lover, but not the other way around. Such a wife must divorce if she wishes to find another companion. A husband seeking to end a marriage will not infrequently simply take up with another woman, forcing his wife to file for the divorce, citing his behavior as the reason—for divorce in Botswana is fault-based.

That Kopano was the one suing for divorce was creating interest, perhaps even sympathy, in the courtroom. Necks were craned to get a better view of the woman who was being divorced for unreasonable behavior. The majority of the people in court were women, and those waiting their turn had stories of abuse, child neglect, adultery, and other sorry tales, all allegedly committed by their husbands. A male story was of great interest, not least because it was rare.

"Can you give the court examples of your wife's unreasonable behavior?" the lawyer asked again.

"She spends a lot of time away from our home. She disappears for weeks, without telling me where she has gone."

The man paused, as if asking that he be excused from saying any more, but his lawyer urged him to go on. She was concerned that he had not placed sufficient grounds before the court for him to be granted divorce.

"She does not love me."

In response to this, a smile played on the wife's lips. Once again

Kopano faltered. The story he finally told, in stops and starts, was that Daisy was in the habit of taking off for weeks on end, without bothering to tell him where she was. He complained that she was inconsiderate and irresponsible. She had taken lovers at various times during their marriage, and his attempts at rebuilding the marriage had failed. He wanted custody of their child, and did not ask that the mother contribute to his support. He also wanted their property to be divided between them. All this, he said, he and his wife had agreed to. He saw no reason for any arguments from his wife, as they had both agreed before the court hearing that she would not contest the divorce.

Indeed, according to court documents signed by the wife, she had agreed to all that her husband was asking for. It was therefore not necessary for her to address the court. Her attendance in court was not even required. She was determined to say her piece, though.

"There is nothing I can say," she started. The court fell silent. She looked up at me, the judge, and her husband from where she was standing, without any trace of fear or embarrassment. When she started to speak, her voice was clear and confident, unlike that of her husband.

"I did not want a divorce. I was hoping that parents could meet."

A sigh escaped Kopano. Weariness enveloped his face. He looked up at his lawyer, his eyes pleading for help.

"May I sit down?" he asked. He sat down and cast down his eyes.

Daisy was a healthy-looking, attractive woman. She was also, obviously, an assertive person, and once she started talking, it was impossible to get her to slow down.

"He is leaving me because I am HIV positive. He is afraid of me. He even locks his door at night as if he is afraid I will come in and give him HIV in his sleep. Our first child fell ill and died. It was a long and painful illness. But we stayed together during all that. The child died of AIDS. It was found out that I too had AIDS. After the child died, my husband was very sad. He wanted another child. He was negative, but he wanted another child. I did not want another child. I was afraid. But he wanted another child. He was very sad."

Daisy paused and her voice faltered slightly before regaining its earlier clarity.

"I gave him the child. I gave him a second child. I was afraid to become pregnant again, but I did. Now I am afraid for this child. I want the child tested. He does not want the child tested."

"My husband is negative. Now he is afraid. I can see his fear in his eyes. At night, when we have to go to bed, I see he is afraid. That is why I sometimes go away; to be with my friends. I drink some wine and I feel better, when I am with my friends. Sometimes I just go and sit with my mother. Day after day, I just sit with her. She doesn't ask questions, and I feel better when I am with her."

Kopano challenged his wife, "Why would I reject you now? I did not reject you when I first found out about your condition."

Daisy cocked her head and shook it slightly, lips pursed before responding. "I even told the doctors, that you are now afraid of me. You are afraid that I will give you AIDS. I say we can use a condom. But you are possessed by fear now. But I do agree that the marriage has broken down. You can have your divorce."

Daisy's public admission that she was HIV positive left the gallery stunned; people sat straight or held tightly to the rails in front of them. After all, the husband had tried to protect her by avoiding the subject.

Even after her concession that the divorce could be granted, Daisy seemed to need to say more, so as the judge I invited the parties to a smaller room where they could have some privacy. After all, the main business of the court had been concluded, the divorce was granted, custody was given to Kopano, and the property—and there was not much—was divided as per their agreement.

"Have you had counseling?" I asked, once we were all seated.

"I have been to counseling, yes. He needs counseling too. But he thinks he can just run and hide away from my AIDS."

Daisy and her now ex-husband were seated on the same two-seater couch. I thought it interesting that in choosing where to sit, they did not try to select seats as far away from each other as possible. That would have been the sort of thing a warring and just-divorced couple would do. I suspected though, that Kopano, had he not been the one to sit down first, would have chosen another seat. He might have thought that he would be considered rude to get up and move to another seat once Daisy had planted herself next to him. He would have noticed too, that the office was not big enough to allow for much choice in seats. He clasped his hands together and stared at them. Daisy raised her head and looked around the office before being brought back by Kopano's words.

"She says I am divorcing her because she has AIDS. That is not true. I stayed with her for a long time even after I knew . . ."

His voice trailed off. His body language suggested extreme fatigue.

A sad smile touched Daisy's lips.

"He is right. When we first found out, he supported me. It was before you could get ARVs from government clinics. They were very expensive, and we had to buy them. I will not lie. He supported me. We bought the ARVs together. We told no one. We would hide as we bought them.

"First our baby was sick. Sick, sick! Have you ever a seen a child so thin he looks like a rope? I would lift that child and her shit would fly across my face. Judge, can you imagine that? I am sorry to use that language, but that is the honest truth. You have never seen a child that sick, dying a little bit every day. We took that child to many doctors, here and in South Africa. I remember a Zulu nurse telling me that only traditional doctors could help. She said, 'My sister, only a *sangoma* can cure this child. What have you done to your ancestors, that this should befall your child?'

"Our families too, were begging us to go to a traditional doctor. They said the child was perhaps bewitched. Or perhaps she was the victim of *dikgaba* [when bad luck follows someone because he or she, or a parent, has done something wrong]. But the two of us, we knew that the child was sick with AIDS. At first we did not know, but then we were told. Am I lying?"

Kopano continued to look down. Daisy continued.

"We were close, during that time. But we were also tired and desperate. We had this secret, that I had AIDS. Those days, a child with AIDS just died. Right in front of your eyes, the child would turn into a listless rope, and the diarrhea! But I will be lying if I say this man did not support me. Remember that he was negative and I was positive and our child was sick. But now he wants to divorce me after all that!"

"But you would disappear for weeks."

"But you knew where to find me. I would go and drink with friends. When I was with my friends, drinking and laughing, I would forget for a little while that I was sick. I could keep the image of my son from my mind. But when I came home, your face said it all. You were not talking to me."

"How was I to know? You would go for days, leaving me with such a young child. You had lovers. I couldn't take it anymore. I was patient for a long time."

"I was sick, and you were beginning to reject me. Don't deny that. You know I would sit with my mother. At first I did not tell her that I had AIDS. Then later, I did, and after that it was so peaceful to sit with her, not talking, but knowing that she supported me."

"Don't forget that you once told me you had another lover! You even told me his name!"

"But you knew I just said that to test you; to make you jealous. You knew."

Kopano shook his head and signed, "Daisy, it's over. This marriage is over."

"I know you still love me. You will come back to me. You are just afraid."

Kopano shook his bowed head and said nothing.

"I just wish you would agree that the child should be tested. Please." Daisy's voice was trembling a bit. Kopano looked up, as if the change in the voice had alarmed him.

"No, not now. If he gets ill, yes. But not now, please." His voice was stronger than before. It was obvious that they were continuing a discussion they had had on many occasions.

"I can't live through another sick child. It would kill me."

"I will take care of this child. This child is okay. He is okay. I have been taking care of him anyway."

"I have agreed to let you have the child. I pray to God that this child is okay."

The couple's story was a sad one, but Daisy was quite a character and while Kopano seemed to prefer silence, she could talk up a storm. By the time they left the office, having agreed to seek counselors and doctors, she had my staff, whose eyes had been teary during the meeting, smiling and on at least two occasions surrendering to bursts of laughter.

"Judge, let me tell you, my life has been sad. You don't want your child to die like mine. I do not wish that on any one. All that flying shit . . . I tell you! Shit can be expensive, I tell you! You run out of disposable nappies and start using only cloth nappies and then you can't keep up with changing the nappies and then shit flies everywhere. I laugh now, because as we say in Setswana, *Leso legolo ke ditshego* [Even the greatest of calamities can induce laughter]. I laugh, but I was not laughing then. I am not laughing in my heart.

"And the lover I told him about, I was just making him jealous. But, of course I did have sex during these years when he was afraid of me. Being sick with AIDS is not medicine against wanting sex. I am still human! Let's not be dishonest here. What was I to do? Can you imagine a man locking the door in your face? What did he expect? That I would rape him? I felt insulted and rejected. I became angry, so of course I had sex with someone else. Hey, I won't say more. I used protection, of course, but I did. What was I to do? I was lonely and my child was dead and I had another one whose status I did not know. What was I to do? He would not even touch me. He wouldn't hold me.

"I did not have a lawyer, but, Judge, I can tell you, this lawyer here was great. I was impossible. She was patient. She was like a mother and sister. She did a great job. She spent hours and hours with us, counseling us. I tell you, I could be impossible. Agreeing to things, then changing my mind. I know the marriage is over, but I am sad that AIDS brought us here.

"But I know he still loves me. *Rra,* you still love me. You will come back to me. I know. You are just afraid of AIDS. But I am happy you didn't get it. That is why I am giving you our son. I know you will look after him. You are not sick, like me. But please, God, I hope he is okay."

❧

Daisy and Kopano are a discordant couple with respect to HIV status. She is HIV infected and he is uninfected. This might seem highly unusual, but it is not. In Botswana, about 20 percent of all stable couples fit this situation, where one spouse or partner is HIV positive and the other is negative. In another 20 percent of couples, both partners are infected, leaving about 60 percent with both uninfected. It may appear that, among discordant couples, it is the woman who is more often infected. But this may be misleading and due to the process by which they are identified. Women are more likely to volunteer for testing and for research trials, and discordant couples are more likely to be identified when an HIV-positive woman is detected and asked if she would like to bring her spouse or male partner for testing as well. Recognizing that numerous people in stable relationships may be HIV positive, the government has now established procedures in many of the testing centers for couples to get tested together.

Obviously, when one partner is infected and the other is not, the positive partner got infected outside the marriage or relationship. In the case of Daisy, this could have happened because she was unfaithful and had sex outside the marriage with an HIV-positive man. It could also have happened during a relationship she had before she was married. As mentioned earlier, the time after infection until an adult develops the signs and symptoms of AIDS is prolonged and variable. We don't know how long after the marriage Daisy and Kopano's first child was born, but we assume it was before Daisy experienced any AIDS-like illness. However, we must also recognize the small possibility that she became infected as a result of her professional activities as a nurse. This is less likely, but possible.

Nurses and physicians sometimes take blood from HIV-positive patients. If they then accidentally stick themselves with a needle and syringe that contains HIV-positive blood, they are at risk of becoming infected. If the skin is just nicked with the needle, the risk is not great. If the plunger goes in and the health care worker is injected with the contaminated blood, the risk is much higher. In any case, someone who is accidentally exposed to HIV-positive blood in this way should immediately begin taking the HAART drug regimen, and continue on the drugs for one month. If the health worker who receives the accidental needle stick starts taking the drugs within twelve hours after exposure, the risk that infection will occur is extremely low. Laboratory researchers who handle HIV to develop vaccines and drugs face this same risk of accidental exposure, and follow the same practice of postexposure prophylaxis if they get cut or stuck with an instrument that contains virus.

Presumably Daisy did not know she was infected when she got married, or when she had her first child, the one who died of AIDS. We are told that she first learned she was infected after her first child developed AIDS. Recognizing that the child could have gotten HIV only from her, she then got tested and realized she also was infected. If she had known she was infected, she probably would have taken drugs to reduce the risk that her child would get infected at the time of birth. It appears that the baby got sick with AIDS at a young age, before HAART therapy was generally available for children. As Daisy says, "Those days, a child with AIDS just died." In Botswana, drug treatment to reduce maternal HIV transmission was available first, two or three years before HAART was widely available to treat clinical AIDS in adults. Treatment for children was not available until at least two or three years after it was available for adults. Even then, it was often available only in the cities, like Gaborone and Francistown.

The impression we have is that Kopano is afraid of becoming infected. This is a natural reaction, particularly when Daisy says they could still have sex if they used condoms, a suggestion he refuses. But then she states that he wanted to have another child. She did not want to, but she agreed to become pregnant again. Surely he must have known that getting her pregnant required them to avoid using condoms and would put him at risk of infection, unless it was done by artificial insemination. Did she receive chemoprophylaxis with AZT or other drugs to reduce the risk that the second baby would be infected? Was she on HAART for her own AIDS illness by then? If so, that would greatly reduce the chance that the second baby would be infected. We are told that they went together to a private physician to get antiretroviral drugs for her own AIDS illness before the drugs were available at government clinics. Kopano doesn't want to get the second child tested for HIV unless the child gets sick. Daisy says that Kopano also needs counseling, and she is right. Daisy also admits that she had sex outside the marriage, after being rejected by Kopano. Did she use condoms in that situation? She said she used protection. If she did not, how could she avoid a pregnancy from the other man, as well as avoid putting him at risk of infection? Did he know she was HIV positive?

With the large number of discordant couples, and a yearning among many of them to have children, what are the options? If the woman is infected and the man is not, he has no risk if he donates sperm and she is impregnated by artificial insemination. It is impossible to eliminate all risk that the infant will become infected, but that risk can be as low as 1 or 2 percent if the pregnant woman is on HAART during the last four or five months of the pregnancy and she does not breastfeed after the baby is born. Having a cesarean section for delivery may reduce the risk to the baby even more. When the man is HIV positive and the woman is not, the situation is also difficult. He can donate sperm, which can then be washed. If this process works correctly, the sperm remain viable; the HIV is in the semen but not in the sperm itself. As an added precaution, the woman can also go on HAART for a month or so, mimicking the type of postexposure prophylaxis that might be followed for a needle stick or a case of rape.

Stigma and discrimination have been associated with HIV testing and disclosure of the infection in many different situations. This is perhaps less likely to be a dominant reaction in situations in Botswana now, during the current stage of the epidemic, when almost all people have a family member or friend who is infected. However, there is still the fear of exposure, and the fear and depression associated with the potential loss of a loved one. Even when patients have a sympathetic and supportive family, they may be reluctant to disclose the situation to others. They know that employers, for example, may be reluctant to retain HIV-positive employees, thinking that they will be less committed to their job, even though extensive evidence indicates that patients receiving adequate antiretroviral therapy usually continue to function just as well as they did before their illness.

In Botswana, the option of testing couples together may lead to opportunities for them to share in treatment and prevention strategies. These might include the use of drugs to reduce transmission in the case of discordant couples, and HAART treatment for both partners if both are positive. At a minimum, it includes shared counseling and education to help plan for family contingencies. Were couples training and counseling available for Daisy and Kopano at the time they realized the first baby was infected?

As rates of HIV infection got very high and the disease began to have an impact on most families, it was inevitable that stigma and discrimination would decrease. Testing to determine HIV infection gradually became more acceptable, especially when people began to realize that drug treatment could save their lives, and could allow those infected to lead productive lives. Perhaps these developments came too late to save the marriage of Daisy and Kopano.

· 3 ·

Masego and Katlego

Mother-to-Child Transmission

MASEGO, THE NIECE OF A FRIEND OF MINE, is twenty-five years old and college educated. She is married to a handsome young man who can be charming and a delight to talk to. They have a beautiful little toddler, a girl. I should say she *was* married, for things have taken a sad turn for the small family.

If this were fifteen years ago, she would be employed, living in a nice house, and perhaps driving her first car. Not now. In the past few years, a college education has not always assured one a job. Since Masego finished college, she has had to depend on temporary jobs and, in between, her mother's support. As for the husband, Katlego, he has only a high school education, so job prospects are even dimmer.

When they met, though, he had a decent job, bringing in a decent income, and there was even a chance that he would be able to buy a stake in the company he worked for. They met in Selebi-Phikwe, far away from each other's sets of friends, so everything was fresh, new, and exciting. In Botswana, with its national population of only 1.7 million people, it is difficult to meet a person about whom you have never heard anything; there is bound to be something that creeps in to spoil the novelty of any new encounter. So it was this seeming newness and freshness that added to the excitement of the love affair. Masego was eager to introduce her new boyfriend to her Gaborone friends, and he was keen to show her the fun part of Selebi-Phikwe. When the temporary job that had taken Masego to Phikwe ended, she stayed on, and when she went home to see her mother, she was always in a hurry to return to Phikwe.

A few months into the relationship, Masego's mother drove into her yard and found the two lovers fighting; punches were being thrown back and forth and Masego was screaming. Masego's mother caught the words.

"You bastard, you have fucked up my life! And now I am pregnant!"

Neither, though, was prepared to say anything to Masego's mother. Masego's mother knew not to pry, for she was well acquainted with Masego's temper. She had been known to throw things when seized by one of her legendary tantrums.

Within months of the fight, however, a wedding was being celebrated; a strong-looking, tall, handsome young man stood next to his seven-months-pregnant new wife. His parents would be hosting the next wedding party the following weekend; the first party was taking place at the bride's house.

"Mmago Cheshe, can you give directions to my sister? She can't find this place. I have tried, but I do not seem to be making myself clear." Nana was my cousin's wife, and she was trying to give directions to her sister, who worked in Jwaneng, where the next wedding party would be. I took the cell phone and gave her directions to where we were.

"Are you sure?"

How can she ask me, am I sure!? No wonder she was not understanding the directions, she was second guessing us instead of listening.

"Yes, turn right at . . ."

A few minutes later Nana's sister arrived, and she seemed to be shaken by something.

"Welcome, I am happy you were able to find the place."

"Oh, my God, Katlego . . ." The woman seemed shocked. From his place at the table I saw Katlego look up, and a look of panic seized his face. He was too far to hear us, though, so I asked, "What is it?"

"Oh nothing, nothing." Still her eyes would not leave the tabletop.

"Do you know him?"

"Oh, a bit. I live in Jwaneng, so we have met."

"But he works in Selebi-Phikwe."

"He has been home a lot. I mean he comes home often."

As I walked away to join the singing, I saw the groom leave his seat and go toward the young woman who had just arrived. I also noticed that the bride was watching them. There were going to be fireworks in the marital bed, I reckoned.

"What was that?" I said to Nana later. "Your sister did not stay long and she seemed shocked to find that Katlego was getting married."

"Well, she says she has known him for a while and had not heard that he was getting married. You know how a marriage gets negotiated over months and word gets out. She was surprised that she had not heard about it, is all."

"You are not telling me the truth."

"Well, Mmago Cheshe, I don't want to be the one to talk about people's secrets."

"Masego saw them speak, and they looked rather suspicious, whispering like that."

"No, it's not like that! My sister works at the hospital. The last time she saw Katlego he was dying! Sick with AIDS! She works in the pharmacy and knows that he and his girlfriend were put on ARVs together only a few months ago. They have a baby! She was surprised to see him well and getting married to someone else! She says some people even believe that he is dead. No one who saw him three months ago would believe all this. She was shocked, really shocked."

A wedding brings together lots of people, and stories get traded and retold and even embellished. Within days, the mysterious handsome man was not so mysterious anymore. The rumor mill churned; he had had a reckless past in Shoshong, he had been jailed once for fraud, he had not one but two children, he had never had a chance of buying himself into the business, he was not to be trusted. Layer upon layer of whispers seeped and spread.

"Masego, you must get tested," Salome, a cousin who was a nurse, advised. She did not say that she was particularly concerned because of what she had heard about Masego's new husband. She was a nurse and she would have given the same advice even if she knew nothing of the whispers about Katlego.

"Yes, I will."

"There is a program for pregnant mothers, the PMTCT program. [PMTCT stands for the prevention of mother-to-child transmission program, which uses ARVs.] It is intended to protect babies from infection."

"I won't breastfeed anyways, so there is no threat to the baby."

"It's more complicated than that. I am not saying you are positive. But if you know, then you will know how to protect your baby. It's best to know."

"I told you I will do it!"

"Okay. But you need to do it soon."

"Why are you on my back? I told you I will do it!"

"I don't have to know. I can refer you to a colleague, if you want."

"Salome, I said I was going to go!"

And she did, and she was found to be positive. She was enrolled in the PMTCT program, and her baby was born negative. She tried to keep the information secret, but with time it was not possible. When it spilled out, it was rather in the same way that her pregnancy had become known, during what had come to be one of many fights with her husband.

"Mmago Cheshe, we are at the police station. Katlego nearly killed my daughter! They were fighting again!"

"Where is she? How is she?"

"She is at the hospital. Her face is all smashed up."

"Where is he?"

"He is here. He has been arrested."

"Where is the baby?"

"At home with the maid. I don't know what would have happened if she had not been there. I am tired of these fights. I am scared something worse is going to happen."

"What were they fighting about?"

"The usual. These people fight all the time. Sometimes she starts it. Sometimes he does. But it's always the same thing! Mmago Cheshe, I can't stand it any more. I am scared something is going to happen!"

"The usual" was a cocktail of frustrations, blame, and cross-blame. Masego was working again, and she, her husband of a few months, and their few-months-old baby girl were living with Masego's mother. Katlego was deeply embarrassed that he and the baby were being supported by a woman. He was particularly embarrassed that they were living with his wife's mother. They could not afford to move out, though; Masego did not make enough to support all three of them. He accused Masego of bossing him around, spending time with her friends and excluding him, and not consulting him on financial issues. Their real life was a far cry from what he had been told it would be by parents and church ministers only a few months before.

"The husband is the head of the family," one of his uncles had said.

"The husband is the head of the family," the church minister had said.

"The husband is the head of the family," one of Masego's uncles had said.

The reality, however, was that he lacked the wits and means to head any family. He had had to surrender his little family to his wife and mother-in-law, and this deeply humiliated him.

Masego, for her part, blamed her husband for infecting her with the HIV virus.

"You bastard, why didn't you tell me?"

"Who says you got it from me? I have asked your friends. You have had lots of boyfriends."

"You were on ARVs and you stopped. I have asked your friends and they have told me! You bastard!"

"You bitch!"

"You live in my mother's house! I feed you and your child!"

"I used to support you. When I worked, I spent all my money on you."

"Well, go out and get a job! I can't support a lazy man."

"I am taking my child to my parents' house. I am not having my child living with my mother-in-law."

"Where will you live?"

"I am coming back right here. I am not letting my wife run around with other men."

"If your child can't live here, how can you?"

"You are selfish. I used to take care of you!"

"Take care of me? You call getting me infected taking care of me?"

"How do you know I infected you?"

"Why didn't you tell me?"

Blame and more blame; fights resulting in injuries; arrests, reconciliations, and more fights.

"Aunty U., I started my ARVs a couple of months ago."

"I hadn't realized that you had been getting ill."

"The doctor said although my viral load was low, the CD4 cell count was also low. They didn't understand."

"What about Katlego?"

"I found out that he was on ARVs at the time we met and then he stopped. He did not want me to find out."

"So he has been off medication for two years?"

"Yes. And when I saw him yesterday, he was not looking well at all."

I did some quick calculations in my head and I began to wonder how Masego could assert as a matter of fact that she had been infected by her husband. Did she really believe that, or was she looking for a scapegoat?

"Aunty U., I can't stay in this marriage. I just can't!"

"Aren't things better? Since you moved out of your mother's house?"

"It's hard for me financially. I have to pay rent, buy food, formula. It's just hard. My mother is helping me, but it's still hard. And I can't cope. If I moved back home, I could cope. And my job! You know how it is. I can never know if I will have it the next month."

"Are you still fighting?"

"Not since I smashed a bottle on his head at Christmas. He knows now that I will fight back. So we only quarrel, but there is no physical violence any more."

"What does he do the whole day?"

"He watches TV and waits to die!"

"What do you mean?"

"Just that. He is waiting to die. You know what he told me the other day? That he will not take ARVs, that he wants to die."

"What do you say to him when he talks like that?"

"What can I say? I have begged him to go see a doctor. I made an appointment for him, but he did not go. I have suggested to him that he go back to school. He had good high school grades, he can still get a government scholarship, he is within the age limit. But he just watches TV the whole day. He has no friends and does not interact with his family."

"Do his parents know he is ill again?"

"How can they know? They don't check on us. I have never seen a family like that."

"If you move back home, he will try to go with you and your mother will not accept that."

"Aunty U., I am tired. I never thought, at my age, I would be where I am. I don't know how I got to this point. I need help."

I heard the "ting" sound, signifying that a text message had just been delivered to my cell phone, and although I had turned the lights off to go to sleep, I turned them back on to read the message. It was from Masego.

"Aunty U., I am going crazy. Please help me."

"What's the matter?" I sent back a text message.

"I need a shrink. I can't cope. I am going crazy!"

"Let me ask around for a suitable person. I will let you know tomorrow."

"Thanks, Aunty U. And thanks for listening to me the other day."

"You're welcome. Good night."

Masego had moved back to her mother's house. Originally it was supposed to be a weekend visit, but when she did not come back home after a night of partying, her mother, on the basis of the past violence between Masego and her husband, had assumed the worst. The police were called, and accusing fingers were pointed at her husband. By the time Masego resurfaced, unharmed and explaining that she had needed time to think, it was clear that the two could not reasonably be expected to live together. The husband had gone back to his home village.

"I hear that Katlego is lying in a room at his parents' house, waiting to die," my sister said to me.

"You spoke to him? What did he say?"

"Yes, before he left I did. I offered to take him to see a doctor. I even offered him a job. He seemed keen but I think he was only fobbing me off."

"He is going to die, unless someone intervenes."

"Mmago Che, did you get my message? I called two days ago." It was Masego's mother calling from Botswana.

"No, I didn't get it. How is everything? Boston is hot!"

"I am afraid I have bad news. Katlego has left us. He died two days ago."

"Oh, my God! Nkamo was saying that he had closed himself up in a house only two weeks ago!"

"Well, he has passed on."

"How is Masego taking it?"

"She is better today. She was really bad two days ago and yesterday."

"Where are you?"

"We are, as is the custom, taking Masego and the girl to Jwaneng. The funeral will be this weekend."

"Give her my condolences."

No doubt Masego will emerge from her husband's funeral torn up about many things. Did she do all she could to save him? Did she drive him to kill himself by accusing him of infecting her? Did he really infect her? After all, she was placed on ARVs within three years of their meeting. Would things have turned out differently if she had considered this other possibility, of being infected by someone else? Her CD4 cell count had to be less than 200 for her to have been put on treatment.

Masego got pregnant, presumably by Katlego, whom she had been going with for some time in Selebi-Phikwe. Within months, a wedding was celebrated—when Masego was seven months pregnant. Masego was from Gaborone, 400 kilometers south of Selebi-Phikwe, where she and Katlego had met. Katlego had formerly been living in Jwaneng and Shoshong, both distant from each other and from Gaborone and Phikwe, so their primary circles of friends and relatives were not known to each other.

When Masego realized that Katlego was infected with HIV, they began to fight. At a wedding celebration, a relative of Masego's realized she knew Katlego, or at least knew about him, in Jwaneng when he was being treated for AIDS. Neither Masego nor her family had known this until recently, but apparently Katlego had had advanced AIDS, and those observing him locally had thought he would die. Masego's relative was amazed to see he seemed to be well and was getting married to someone who was already pregnant.

Patterns of behavior that involve unprotected sex with multiple concurrent partners may be particularly dangerous for HIV transmission. In a pattern sometimes referred to as grazing, a man may have partners in different sites, or "multiple houses." Having multiple concurrent relationships seems to be riskier than multiple consecutive relationships.

Katlego had apparently been successfully treated for AIDS with antiretroviral drugs, to the point where he felt well and resumed a vigorous life that included sexual relationships. After being on ARVs for some time, many AIDS patients recover from their symptoms and want to return to normal activities, including sex. When beginning treatment, most patients have very high amounts of HIV in their body and release the virus in semen or vaginal fluids, thereby infecting their partners. When they are on steady courses of ARV drugs, viral loads drop dramatically and the risk of infecting sex partners is much lower. But some risk is always there. It is unclear whether Katlego had stopped taking the drugs when he became involved with Masego, thus increasing the risk that she would be infected, or whether he was still taking the drugs without her knowledge (and without her having the knowledge that he was indeed HIV infected). So was Masego infected by Katlego? Perhaps, but this is by no means certain.

The relative who discovered that Masego's new husband was the Katlego she had known in Jwaneng also apparently knew that both he and a previous girlfriend were being treated for AIDS—another girlfriend with whom he had a baby.

Upon learning all this, Masego was obviously confused and distressed about her own situation and that of the baby she was carrying. A baby is most likely to be infected when the mother has a high amount of virus—a high viral load (VL)—in her body. A high VL may be up to 100,000 viruses per drop of blood. In most instances, a high VL is present for several weeks after initial infection—called the acute phase—and then it drops down to a low level for a few years—the set point—owing to the temporary success of the body's own immune response in controlling the infection. After a few years the immune response starts to fail, with the HIV winning the battle against the human body, and VL gradually goes back up. The key cells involved in immune control lose out and fall to a few hundred per milliliter of blood. At this point an infected person again becomes more infectious to his or her sex partners, and soon after, he or she often develops clinical signs and symptoms of AIDS.

Infants may become infected before birth, during the process of birth, and after birth if breastfeeding occurs. Masego is right in assuming that the baby will not be infected after birth if she does not breastfeed. However, she is very wrong if she believes that the baby can be infected only by breastfeeding after birth. In fact the risk of infection may be even higher before birth, during the last months of pregnancy, and when the baby is passing through the birth canal. Thus, if Masego does not begin taking chemoprophylaxis drugs immediately after learning she is HIV positive, when she is already seven months pregnant, the baby is at great risk of becoming infected before birth. If that happens, avoiding breastfeeding will do no good. The virus in southern Africa appears to be especially effective at infecting before birth, and the best approach to blocking such fetal transmissions is to begin chemoprophylaxis earlier, at twenty-eight weeks of pregnancy or before. At more than seven months pregnant, Masego is already a bit beyond this stage.

Although the infant can be infected before birth, it is also at particularly high risk while passing through the birth canal. In instances where antiretroviral drugs cannot be given during pregnancy, especially before the seventh or eighth month of pregnancy, one drug—nevirapine (NVP)—is often given alone to the mother at the onset of labor, and then to the newborn infant. This has been found to reduce by up to half the number of neonatal infections that would otherwise occur. Drugs other than NVP do not seem useful for stopping neonatal infections unless administration is begun at least one to two months earlier, before birth.

Sometimes, particularly in rural areas, pregnant women do not present themselves to midwives or other health officials until they go into labor. When beginning to take NVP at this stage, half or more of the mothers who receive it rapidly develop a resistance to the drug. This poses substantial complications for them in the future, as NVP resistance in the mother may then persist for at least six months. If the mother then becomes severely ill with AIDS—a more likely possibility if she had a very high VL during childbirth and was more likely to infect the infant—she will need AIDS disease treatment with highly active antiretroviral therapy. One of the three drugs routinely used in combination for HAART is NVP. If a mother is already resistant to NVP, HAART treatment often fails. And if she cannot be adequately treated, she dies and leaves her infant without a mother.

In most African cultures women routinely breastfeed their infants, and before AIDS they had been encouraged to do so by international health agencies such as the World Health Organization (WHO), because of the nutritional benefits to the baby. At the entrance to Livingstone Hospital in Molepolole, Botswana, a sign was posted stating BREAST IS BEST. In the era of AIDS in Africa, however, breastfeeding may be dangerous unless the HIV-positive mother is on HAART, which greatly reduces levels of HIV in both her blood and her milk. Masego, as a college-educated working woman, may feel somewhat less pressured to breastfeed, relieving her of some of the stigma and humiliation that might be felt by young women who are not fully employed. Women who use formula rather than breastfeeding may feel stigmatized in many situations in Africa.

Under normal circumstances, breast milk is the best source of nutrition for the infant, and it also provides some protective antibodies for immunity against diarrhea and pneumonia, which babies are prone to get—especially when receiving fluids such as formula that may be made with contaminated water or unclean utensils, or given in unsterilized bottles. Even breastfeeding women who are HIV infected can still pass on some immune protection against other childhood diseases, but certainly none to offset the risk of getting HIV. And those other infections can often, though not always, be eliminated with the right antibiotics. In most places in Botswana, drinking water is generally safe, but this may not always be the case in rural sites; flooding from unusually heavy rainfall may also contaminate water sources. In many African countries, pure water is not ordinarily available.

Numerous studies are under way to determine how to lower the risk of HIV infection in infants as well as lower the other causes of disease and death in infants who are born to HIV-positive mothers. One approach is to administer ARVs to the pregnant woman as early as possible before delivery. Often the drugs and even the drug combinations are the same as those given to patients with active AIDS disease; they are given to HIV-positive pregnant women even when they seem to be healthy. Ongoing trials are testing different combinations of the drugs, different start times for administering them, and different methods to assure that the drugs are taken. Success in taking the drugs is obviously related to convenience, cost, and availability, as well as to the side effects that some may cause, like vomiting and diarrhea. Some anti-HIV drugs have been contraindicated during pregnancy because of the risk that the drug itself may cause fetal defects, but most appear safe for the developing fetus.

Another category of research is targeted at reducing those infant HIV infections that occur during the process of birth. This becomes imperative when the woman discovers that she is HIV positive only when tested near the time of delivery. In some cases at this stage, an HIV infection has already been established in the infant. But a large fraction of the "birth infections" could be prevented with at least one drug, nevirapine. As mentioned above, this treatment does raise the problem of NVP resistance in the mother, and in those infants who may already have become infected in the womb. An essential drug that may be needed later for the mother and her infant is then lost as a disease treatment option, at least for a while. Cesarean sections have been shown to significantly reduce birth infections with HIV, yet obviously this is an option only when skilled surgery personnel and sterile equipment are available.

A third area of research is under way to determine how best to retain the benefits of breastfeeding while reducing milk-related infant infections. One approach involves early weaning, with supplementation using a high-protein gruel called *tsabana* after three or four months, when the more unique benefits of milk-related nutrition and antibodies are largely gone. This, however, does not eliminate the risk from nursing right after birth, nor does it eliminate the stigma that may be attached to early cessation of breastfeeding. Studies have shown that HIV infection by breastfeeding can be a risk for many months, up to at least two years, so eliminating much of the breastfeeding period can be beneficial. Another approach is to allow the baby to breastfeed, but to give prophylactic drugs to the baby at the same time, to reduce or block the establishment of HIV. This follows the same rationale behind giving drugs in advance of a positive HIV diagnosis to medical workers who accidentally get stuck with a needle containing HIV-positive blood, or to rape victims who may have been assaulted by a man who was HIV-positive.

Still another approach that is very effective is to provide extensive drug therapy to all HIV-positive mothers while they are breastfeeding. Just as the drug treatment dramatically lowers virus levels in the blood, it has also been shown to lower virus levels in breast milk (as well as in reproductive fluids), thus greatly reducing the amount of virus that the baby might receive by breastfeeding. Various other approaches have been suggested, such as having HIV-infected mothers pump their breast milk and then pasteurize it before feeding it to the baby. But many such interventions are clearly not practical, especially in developing regions of the world. The careful use of combinations of available options can reduce infant infections by at least 90 percent, from approximately 2 in 5 infants that might be infected by their mother in the absence of any intervention, to about 1 in 50 or 100.

Very recent research results indicate that even breastfeeding mothers can reduce infant transmission rates to 1 to 2 percent if they take three-drug HAART combinations beginning by month six of pregnancy, and continue taking the drugs while breastfeeding. Progress in safe methods to greatly reduce infections has been one of the bright spots in AIDS research as it relates to sub-Saharan Africa. Sadly, the lack of adequate public health leadership, infrastructure, trained personnel, and resources has greatly delayed the implementation of such measures to prevent infant infections in most countries. However, Botswana has been proactive in implementing such programs, and about 90 percent of pregnant women get tested and then receive drugs to reduce transmission if they are HIV positive.

Masego's baby was presumably not infected when tested soon after birth. In the absence of breastfeeding, if the baby was not infected by one month of age (from transmission in childbirth or during the pregnancy), the baby is at virtually no risk of being infected until he or she is an adolescent and becomes sexually active. Although people at any age could be infected through injections with contaminated blood, such as with unscreened transfusions or the illicit use of contaminated needles, this should be very rare, especially in children, except in unusual situations where they may have anemia due to malaria or trauma.

Testing the infant or young child to confirm the absence of infection, however, is not as easy as testing adults. Along with protective antibodies to diarrheal bacteria that the infant gets from the mother in breast milk, antibodies to HIV are also transmitted to the infant, even when HIV itself is not. And while such antibodies act as a surrogate marker for infection in adults, they cannot be used as such a measure in children, at least not until the child is a year or two old. Until then, a more complicated and expensive test, the polymerase chain reaction (PCR), must be used, and this test is not available except in more advanced laboratories. Determining whether young infants are actually infected or are just giving a false-positive reaction is not possible in less developed rural areas.

After some time has passed, Masego herself starts on HAART drugs for her own illness. Although it isn't clear how sick she has become, the doctor said her CD4 cell count was low. In all areas of the world, it is recommended that patients go on HAART therapy if their CD4 count falls below 200. In Botswana this level is now set at 250, and in the United States and Europe it is 350. Treatment is recommended at these levels even if the patients are not yet visibly sick. If the CD4 count falls much lower, there is concern that disease and death could occur very rapidly, or that the immune system could not be resurrected by the antiretroviral drugs. And once therapy for AIDS begins, the patient should remain on therapy for life. As with high blood pressure or diabetes, the disease is not cured, so the patient cannot stop treatment. It is only kept under control.

That Masego apparently needed therapy within a few years after she met Katlego actually increases the possibility that she was initially infected by someone else, in an earlier relationship. Although clinical AIDS can arise within a year or two after infection, this is unusual. Ordinarily people do not develop clinical AIDS or severe immune system destruction (i.e., a CD4 count below 200) in less than three or four years after infection. Usually it takes six to eight years.

Why Katlego died at the time he did is also confusing. He seemed to give up taking the drugs, choosing to die rather than live with continuing guilt and despair. However, the HAART drugs sometimes have severe side effects, causing nausea, vomiting, diarrhea, and various other forms of severe discomfort. In Katlego's case, he may have stopped taking the drugs when he began living with Masego simply to hide the fact that he had HIV/AIDS. Or, like some patients, he may have decided that the treatment is as bad as the disease and stopped taking his medication. Even sporadic periods of going off the medication cause drug resistance to develop much more rapidly. When a patient goes back on the same drugs, or even related drugs, they no longer have the same health-restoring benefits. Increasing numbers of new drugs that do not share the same "cross-resistance" are becoming available, but they are usually much more expensive and require more expensive monitoring and more sophisticated lab tests, as well as highly skilled and experienced health care personnel.

Death may always seem to be unfair, but it seems especially so when the victim is young. When deeply linked to sexual activity, procreation, and even the processes of birth and breastfeeding, the transmission of death by HIV seems particularly cruel.

Mandla Gets Tested

Diagnosis of HIV Infection

"JUDGE DOW, MANDLA IS ILL. Please talk to him. Please, Judge. You helped me. Help him." Lucy has been on therapy now for about a year, and to look at her you would never believe she was ever close to death. She has now made it her business to drag anyone who looks ill to my office, demanding that I talk to them.

Mandla, the young man Lucy was talking about, was in his mid-thirties, and until recently he had been an athletic-looking man. He was tall and broad shouldered with an easy if somewhat shy smile. He worked in the criminal registry and because not infrequently the system failed, he was always shyly but firmly trying to get one judge or another to accept yet one more file to be listed in their roll. His gentle demeanor always won with me, and his gratitude, whenever I agreed to hear a case he had failed to list, was always genuine. I was therefore keen to see how I could help, but I was also apprehensive since I knew that Lucy, the self-appointed HIV/AIDS police-woman, would not be urging me to see Mandla if there were nothing to it.

After days of ducking and dodging, Mandla was seated across from me in my office, and his broad shoulders appeared even broader and his neck appeared dry and sticklike. He kept on rubbing a pen between his large hands. He was nervous and looked everywhere except at me.

"Judge, my problem is that I drink too much on weekends. I am not ill, really, I am not, Judge. Too much beer has always given me diarrhea. Sometimes, I mean. Not always. Only sometimes."

"Are you drinking any more than you have been in the past years?"

"Well, no, Judge. No really, the reason why I am ill is that I work in a cold room. That office is cold and dusty. It can make any one ill. I get chills and when people see me using a heater they just assume I have AIDS!"

"Mandla, you know that Lucy was very ill only last year?"

"Yes, Judge. I don't want to talk about her private matters."

"You know she is the one who has insisted that I talk to you?"

"Yes. I know the rumors. That she has AIDS. That is her business. People talk too much."

"How many death notices have you seen this year alone? How many times have you contributed to someone's funeral this year alone?" Every time someone from the judicial offices died, a notice was circulated and everyone had to contribute a bit of money, which would then be delivered to the family by those staff members who attended the funeral. There had been so many death notices in the past three years that many employees had begun to complain that they could not keep up with the contributions.

"Judge, you know if it's someone's time, it's their time. No one can dodge death."

"You saw Lucy, when I first took her to the hospital? You were there." I remembered he had been among the people who had watched as others had helped me carry Lucy to the car after she had collapsed in the key room.

"Yes, yes. But Judge, honestly, if I stop drinking and eat well, I will be fine. I just had problems at home. You know how it is. You start doing well at work and then bad things start happening to you. Even if you don't believe in witchcraft you can see bad things coming your way. I tell you, Judge—"

"Mandla, don't you think knowing what is the matter with you would be a good start?"

"What is the point of knowing that you are going to die? We are all going to die at one point. What is the point of knowing when?" His thin chin was pointed stubbornly at me and he was facing me for the first time since he had come into the room.

"But you do not have to die! Not any more. Look at Lucy."

"I will have to think about it." He licked his dry, blistering lips and I could see fear in his eyes.

"I can go with you. To test, I mean. If that will make it easy for you."

"I have a child. I will have to think about it."

An hour later, Mandla left my office and Lucy shot in. "Did he agree to test? Judge, did you persuade him?" When I told her that Mandla had promised to think about testing, she was not satisfied. "You have to try again. Otherwise he will die. Did you tell him that he will surely die if he does not get tested and get help?"

I knew that Lucy's assessment was not an exaggeration. Mandla was losing weight fast, and he had blisters spotting his lips and admitted to having had bouts of diarrhea. All he needed was the onset of some serious illness or even repeated bouts of diarrhea, and his condition would slide closer to death.

For the next few weeks Mandla and I went over the same ground without his budging from his position that he was thinking about it. Once he accompanied me to the local counseling and testing center for a reconnaissance visit. He had made it clear that he was not ready to test but wanted to go to observe what kind of people went there and to find out what kind of questions were asked by the counselors.

Seeing how anxious he was, I wondered, not for the first time, whether the center was the best place for him to do the test. The process, it seemed to me from past experiences, was too theatrical and bore no resemblance to what happened at "normal" hospital visits. First comes the counseling, which involves detailed questions about one's sex life, including number of partners and the last sexual encounter and whether condoms were used or not. Then follow questions about what result you expect, whom you will tell in the case that you are positive, whether you have the person's phone number ready, whether you checked that he or she will be available to take your call. Then you are quizzed about how prepared you are for a positive result. By this time you might wonder whether you should leave the room. Then a silver metal bowl with a lid is brought in. You are told that your test result will come in that bowl and that you will be the person to take off the lid and read the result for yourself. You are told how to read the result—that two bars means positive and one bar means negative. Then you are declared counseled and ready to take the test, and once again you are asked if you still wish to continue. Even the most determined of persons may be excused for deciding to slip out the main door upon leaving the counseling room, instead of going through with the test.

Assuming that you stay on to have blood taken, and wait for the twenty or so minutes it takes for the reaction, the drama with the silver bowl can be too much for some. You are once again led back to the counseling room, the lidded silver bowl is brought in and placed on the table in front of you, you are asked if you still remember what two bars means and what one bar means, you are asked if you are sure. By this time you might not be sure anymore. You might ask to be reminded, and that will be done. You are asked once again if you are certain about your expectation and whether you are ready for a positive result. In the meantime, the silver bowl is sitting between you and the counselor, ominously waiting to reveal its contents.

Finally, you are asked to remove the lid, and when you do, when you face the one bar or two bars, you are asked what the result means!

I was not sure that Mandla could deal with all that drama. In fact I knew of someone who, having gone through the whole process, left the room after the silver-bowl presentation phase. He says that first he refused to take off the lid, insisting that that was the job of the nurse. After some argument the nurse obliged, but then, when faced with the result, he could not remember whether it was two bars or one bar that meant a positive status, and when the counselor insisted that he be the one to interpret the result, he argued otherwise. It ended in a stalemate and he stormed out of the room.

"But what was your result? Was it two bars or one bar?" I asked.

"How am I to know? Do I look like a nurse?"

"I have had the test, so if you tell me, I can tell you your status."

"Mmago Cheshe, I don't remember! I went to those people for them to tell me whether I have the virus or not. Not to be taught to be a doctor! If I wanted to know if I had a broken leg, were they going to ask me to read the X-ray sheet?"

He might have had a few beers by the time we had this conversation, but I thought that he had a point. Even if I persuaded Mandla to test, a prospect that did not seem likely, he might still pull out before the process was complete.

I continued to discuss the importance of testing with Mandla, giving examples of people I knew who had benefited from it, but Mandla did not seem close to changing his mind. I was about to give up when he burst into my office one lunch break and announced, with a smile that exposed his beautiful teeth and somehow overshadowed his still blistering lips, "Judge, I have tested. I have tested! Thank you! I have tested!"

"Oh, that's good." I was relieved that I was wrong about his status but was already wondering what then could be wrong with him, for although his elation was giving him a bounce, there was no doubt that he was sick with something.

"I am positive." He said it so firmly and with such jubilation that I thought he meant the opposite.

"Oh."

"Yes, I am positive. I tested and I was told I have the virus. Thanks, Judge. Just knowing is such a burden from my shoulders. Now I can start treatment. I have been referred to a clinic in Gaborone and soon I can start treatment. I called my girlfriend. She is on her way right now with our baby. They, too, are going to test today. I have been talking to her for weeks, and today I just decided to grab the bull by the horns and test!"

Within days it seemed like Mandla had told almost everyone at the office about his status.

"You won't believe what that chap in the registry told me today. Out of the blue he told me that he is positive and that he is starting ARVs soon. I thought that was brave, telling me just like that!" Judge W. announced at tea one Friday. Little did he know of the mental anguish that Mandla had been through.

❖

The testing that is done to determine whether adults are infected with HIV does not check directly for the virus; rather, it checks for the presence of antibodies that have been produced by the body in response to the infection. Sites that provide HIV testing and counseling, called Tebelopele centers in Botswana, are located throughout the country and in most other countries in Africa. The cost of the test is minimal, only a dollar or two, and there are other modest costs for the needle and syringe to take the blood and the personnel to collect the blood, interpret the results, and provide counseling to the client. The accuracy of the test is extremely high. False positives and false negatives can occur, but they are very rare. When a test result is hard to interpret, a repeat test is done with a new blood sample taken a few weeks later and the result is readily resolved.

Tests that use saliva rather than blood are also available. They are slightly less accurate than the blood tests, and are usually used only for epidemiologic surveys to estimate the proportion of a particular population that might be infected. If, for example, a mining company needs to estimate the number of its employees that may be HIV infected, more workers may be willing to provide saliva by spitting in a cup than to be stuck with a needle to obtain blood.

The tests for diagnosing HIV infection with antibodies are highly sensitive and specific, with two exceptions. The first exception is for adults who were infected within the last two to four weeks before testing, too recently to have developed the antibodies. At this stage a flulike acute febrile illness is often present, but not always. If such an individual tests negative, a different type of test can be tried, the polymerase chain reaction or PCR test, which detects the genes of HIV. This test is similar in design to those used in forensic medicine to detect DNA from a suspected criminal at a crime site. Alternately, simply testing again for antibodies a month or two later will give an accurate result.

The second exception is for infants under eighteen months of age, when maternal antibodies are still in their system. All infants born to HIV-positive mothers acquire passively transmitted maternal antibodies—including HIV antibodies, whether or not they in fact have HIV; those who are not infected with the virus will appear as false positives on the antibody test. Again, the PCR test will immediately reveal whether the child is actually infected.

HIV antibody tests are done on about 10,000 people in Botswana every year to get an estimate of the number of people in the country who are infected. Most recently this testing led to estimates that about 24 percent of adults in Botswana are infected. A door-to-door survey produced an estimate that about 18 percent of the population is infected, when children (who have lower rates of infection) are included with adults.

The annual national survey tests, as well as employee tests done at places of work, are usually done in an anonymous way. For Mandla, of course, the test is a personal choice, to determine if he is infected. As he is already showing symptoms—diarrhea, weight loss, and lip blisters—the positive HIV test also serves as a definitive diagnosis for AIDS disease. It is interesting that Lucy, one of Mandla's co-workers, had been through a similar experience, even collapsing at work and being carried out for emergency treatment. After she tested positive and was successfully treated with HAART, she became a strong advocate for testing and counseling. This illustrates how the availability of antiretroviral drugs can serve as an important stimulus for people to learn whether they are infected. Knowing they are positive may lead to a better life, if treatment is available and successful, as is usually the case in Botswana.

It is assumed that widespread testing and counseling will lead to lower numbers of new infections. This may be true to some extent because people who know they are infected may not want to put uninfected loved ones at risk through unprotected sex—or untreated pregnancy, in the case of pregnant women. Also, there is good evidence that treatment with HAART drugs greatly decreases the amount of virus in reproductive fluids, decreasing the chance of infection through sexual contact even when protective means, such as condoms, are not used. Experimental trials are currently under way in Botswana and a few other countries to see if the treatment of HIV infections using HAART in an infected spouse will diminish the risk of transmission to an uninfected spouse. The same approach might be tested in entire villages or towns, by examining whether the use of HAART for all HIV-positive people who are most likely to infect others lowers the rate of new infections in the entire community.

In trying to induce Mandla to get himself tested, Judge Dow reminds him about the numerous death notices that he has seen and how often he has contributed to the cost of a funeral. It is a standard cultural practice in Botswana for large gatherings of relatives and friends to participate in prolonged funeral sessions. The friends of the deceased are invited to contribute to the expenses, as the funeral is associated with a large meal and the family of the deceased may be destitute because they exhausted all financial resources in taking care of the member who has slowly died of AIDS.

The testing experience that Mandla went through is traumatic, with questions about sexual practices and who should be notified about the results. After the questioning, and before the actual test, Mandla was asked if he wanted to continue. In fact, many people who go in for HIV tests—whether for personal diagnosis, public health surveys, or for participation in research trials—fail to return for their results. When HIV tests were first available, they usually took hours or even days to process, increasing the chances that clients would not return for their results. In recent years, "rapid tests" have become more accurate and more accessible, decreasing the chance that a client will change his or her mind about wanting to know the result. While fear of a positive result is understandable, the reaction of relief expressed by Mandla after his testing represents the first step toward recovery from the debilitation of clinical AIDS.

· 5 ·

The Death of Mma Monica

AIDS Disease in Adults and Availability of Treatment

MMA MONICA DIED on the thirteenth of January, 1997, surrounded by aunts. At least five at any one time had been with her, had bathed her twice a day, run a cold cloth across her body constantly, and turned her creaking bones as often as they could bear her groans of pain. At least five times a day, a liquid mixture of porridge and water had been poured down her throat. Her mouth had to be pried open, forcing her clenched teeth apart. Her eyes had swiveled around the room, refusing their entreaties that she close them and rest.

The skeleton that was the dying Mma Monica lay on a mattress on the floor; the bed had long been removed to another room to allow easy access to her. The aunts-in-waiting occasionally, perhaps to distract themselves, discussed such mundane matters as the fact that the rains had been bad, and the preference for loud music among the young. Generally though, they were quiet, watching the rise and fall of Mma Monica's chest for signs of the final surrender. They had started to speak openly about that prospect and how it was the only way out of the pain.

Outside the bedroom, one of three in the five-room house, at least three more aunts sat, waiting for their turn to help. The topics of their discussions, although always veering toward the limited prospects for Mma Monica's recovery, were more wide ranging. They discussed the grandchildren they had left at home, the scourge of death sweeping through the country, and failed crops; they lamented the plummeting waistlines of their daughters' jeans. Occasionally a groan of pain from the bedroom would stop a sentence midtrack. Then an inquiry would be made as to whether anything new needed to be done, or a silence would ensue. Inside and outside the bedroom, their waiting was for one thing only, death.

Outside the house, under the mulberry tree, a group of uncles were chatting in subdued voices; they, too, were waiting for only one thing—death. They, too, had been meeting daily, for at least two weeks, under that tree—that is, since word was sent out by the nursing aunts that the only reliever of pain for Mma Monica would be death. A neighbor had mercifully provided a bucket of traditional beer so the uncles, and an aunt or two, could drown a bit of the sorrow as they waited for the inevitable.

In the cooking area a few meters from the uncles, young women were preparing yet another meal for the uncles and the aunts. Young women had been coming to Mma Monica's home for weeks; there were enough of them to work on a rotational basis, and they too were subdued. They too were waiting for the inevitable.

Mma Monica's three daughters were lying down in one of the bedrooms. Occasionally one of them, red-eyed and fatigued, ventured out to the waiting aunts to find out if there was anything new.

"How is she?"

"Nothing has changed, my child. Go and lie down. There is nothing any one can do now. We have to wait for her to surrender so the pain will end."

"Can I see her?"

"It will only bring pain to your heart, my child. Nothing has changed."

"Let her go in and see her. That is the only way she can accept the inevitable," another aunt advised.

"Okay, my child. Go in. But have a strong heart."

The daughter was met, yet again, by her mother's swiveling eyes. Was her mother trying to tell her something? She seemed so alive behind those eyes! The daughter took the face towel from one of the aunts, dipped it in cold water, wrung it out and ran it over her mother's forehead. She wanted to ask why they were feeding her if they were all waiting for her death. She wanted to question why the Catholic sisters had seemed to be unclear about exactly what they were praying for; was it for her mother's recovery or her death? She wanted to protest that it was this confusion about their wishes and hopes that had locked her mother in the impasse between life and death.

"Our Father, who art in Heaven, release this child of God from suffering and receive her soul, if that be thy will," one sister had prayed.

"It is within your power, oh Lord, for full recovery to be restored to this ailing friend of ours. Have mercy and give her strength," yet another had prayed.

She was afraid to confront what *she* wished for, especially after she had observed her mother being bathed with soil from her ancestral birthplace, the indication that, so far as her aunts and uncles were concerned, the only way out of the pain for her mother was death. How could there be any return from this point? How could life possibly be breathed into the skeletal form that was her mother; how could those lips ever be pulled sufficiently to cover those bared teeth?

Mma Monica had been sick, at first on and off, for at least five years. During that time, until the last year, she had always been able to recover enough to go back to work. When she was attacked by a bad flu, she was able to rise from her bed, and after a while no one remembered that she had been ill. When she had a bout of diarrhea she had gone to the local hospital, and within days she was back to a good semblance of her earlier self. When she had the attacks of blisters around her lips, she slapped on some gentian violet and things seemed to get back to normal after some weeks. Then she had an attack of pimples, and swollen lumps behind her ears, and she joked that she was having both childhood mumps and teenage acne at the same time. All the time though, little by little, Mma Monica was losing weight. At first it was not even noticeable, until one day an old friend made the observation out loud, and Mma Monica retorted angrily that she too could say some things about the friend that were obvious but unattractive. Everyone listening was shocked by her angry outburst; later, when the conversation was recalled, it was accepted that she must have known then that she had the unmentionable disease.

During the years of her decline, even until a week before her death, Mma Monica had tried everything in her attempt to meet the HIV monster eating her up. She had gone to the hospital, only to find out that, except for treating the opportunistic infections, there was nothing that could be done for her. At first no one had seemed prepared to name what was ailing her, but finally the doctor had told her; her problem stemmed from what she had done years ago; she had had unprotected sex with an HIV-infected partner.

She had gone to not one but a total of three churches, which all suggested that if she believed enough she would be cured. At one of the churches she had been bathed in holy water, with holy men dancing around her and entreating the bad spirits to leave her diseased body. Her problem, it was said, stemmed from her limited belief in the power of the Lord.

She had gone to a traditional doctor, who, having cast his bones, diagnosed her problem as stemming from her jealous sentiments toward a work colleague. If only she could purge her heart of these bad tendencies. A batch of medicines was prescribed, but it really lay within her to cure her illness.

She went to a spiritual healer, who bit into her chest and sucked the disease out. She saw, with relief, the *sejeso*—a creature that grows inside the body, causing disease—quivering in a bloody blob at her feet and believed herself to be cured. A month later, when her health had not improved, she was back at the healer's place, where she learned the removal had not been successful; tentacles of the *sejeso* had broken off and had since grown back into a full creature. More powerful forces were resisting her curing. Had she perhaps annoyed an uncle, an aunt?

And except for that one doctor at the hospital, no one was naming the monster within her; not the nurses, not her relatives, not her friends—and certainly she was not, herself.

The nurses wrote in code on her medical card, so neither she nor anyone else could understand what they had written of "this disease," "the new disease," "the radio disease," "the disease with no cure." To the traditional doctors and the spiritual healers, she was either bewitched or receiving her just deserts for bewitching someone herself.

The recurring message was clear, though: she was going to die. And they all had to be telling the truth. All around her, work colleagues, friends, and relatives were dying.

By the time she surrendered to her death at around noon that January in 1997, the sighs escaping the lips of those around her were of relief. For days they had waited for the mercy of the final sleep. Not one had ever named aloud the monster in the room.

❖

In 1997, when Mma Monica died, the antiretroviral drugs that could have saved her life were not available in Africa. They were already available in Europe and America, but they were very expensive, and at that time little thought had been given to making them available in Africa. Most of the drugs were under patents controlled by the pharmaceutical companies, and it was believed that only physicians who were experienced specialists were capable of administering the drugs and monitoring their patients' progress. Just a tiny fraction of the physicians then seeing AIDS patients in Africa had experience with ARVs. The cost of the drugs was estimated to be in the tens of thousands of dollars per year of life, not something that could be imagined for Africa, where the median income was a few hundred dollars per year. Even in Botswana, one of the wealthier countries thanks to its diamond mines, mean income might be a few thousand dollars per year. This was way below the levels needed to purchase the drugs, and there was obviously a complete lack of experienced medical personnel who knew how to administer the drugs.

By 2001 or 2002, a small number of Africans began to receive AIDS drugs from a few entrepreneurial private practitioners. But they often received only one or two drugs, rather than the best combinations of three drugs that were widely used in the rich countries. This resulted in high rates of drug resistance and clinical failure, similar to the situation in the United States in the late 1980s or early 1990s before the three-drug HAART combinations were available. By 2004 or 2005, however, everything would change in Botswana. By 2002, the government of Botswana had made block purchases of the three-drug combinations needed for HAART treatment, and large numbers of physicians and nurses were being rapidly trained to give the drugs, through a Harvard University program of short courses sponsored jointly by the Gates Foundation and the Merck Foundation. By 2005, numerous AIDS treatment centers were bustling all over the country. At the Princess Marina Hospital in Gaborone, about 15,000 AIDS patients were being treated, probably the largest number of AIDS patients treated at a single facility anywhere in the world.

The treatment program was associated with much good news. The lives of most patients were saved, even those as severely ill as Mma Monica. The expansion and success of the medical treatment was accompanied by a profound depression of the funeral industry, but the rest of the economy seemed to be expanding again. Those patients who were treated regained their health and vigor and returned to work. It seemed that eventually the program would pay for itself. The cost of antiretroviral drugs plummeted as low-cost generics began to be produced. And the population that would otherwise have been lost to AIDS, mostly young adults who had already acquired most of their education and life skills, would be able to continue working and repay society for this investment.

Remarkably, or so it seemed at the time, success rates for treatment of AIDS patients in Botswana were just as good as those seen at the major medical centers in the United States and Europe. It was soon apparent that some of the less expensive antiretroviral drug combinations worked very well, and also that nurses and physicians with less extensive training could have good success. Rigorous adherence to a schedule of taking the drugs at regular intervals was also known to be extremely important, as missed doses greatly increased the chance that drug-resistant viruses would emerge. But patients in Africa were generally very conscientious about sticking to schedules, even when taking the drugs sometimes caused side effects like nausea.

When the first patients received antiretroviral drugs in Botswana in late 2001 or 2002 through the public system, battlefield-type triaging was practiced and the most severely ill patients were treated first. As the medical system caught up with the number of patients, more and more were treated before they became debilitated. As of 2008, HIV/AIDS patients in Botswana received HAART treatment when their immune system dropped to 250 CD4 lymphocytes per cubic millimeter of blood. When treated at this level, 90 percent or more survive, go back to work, and resume living a normal life. Although the HIV will never be eliminated from the body, it can be managed with drugs in much the same way that high blood pressure and insulin-dependent diabetes are managed.

Even patients as severely ill as Mma Monica was in 1997 may recover with HAART and careful support therapy. Although her CD4 cells were probably almost all gone, with perhaps only 10 to 50 per cubic millimeter remaining, significant immune restoration may occur with proper therapy.

The symptoms shown by Mma Monica are typical for AIDS in Africa—the general malaise, fever, and respiratory symptoms often called a flulike syndrome: chronic diarrhea, swollen lymph nodes, herpes fever blisters, and chronic weight loss, or "wasting." The wasting is largely due to a loss of appetite associated with fever and malaise, but a resulting metabolic syndrome then accelerates the loss of weight. Although general antibiotics or drugs for TB may provide some delay before the most severe symptoms, only antiretroviral HAART can reverse the process.

The year Mma Monica died, 1997, was at the beginning of the major wave of disease and death from AIDS in Botswana. Because the epidemic of infection had just begun to expand in about 1990 and did not reach peak infection rates until about 1997, the peak time for disease from AIDS would be in 2004 or 2005, right when HAART treatment was becoming widely available.

The availability of treatment might be expected to affect rates of HIV testing in multiple ways. For example, many might be more willing to be tested for HIV if they knew it could lead to treatment to save their life. In the early days of the HIV epidemic in the United States, before ARV drugs were available, it was difficult to get high-risk homosexual men to get tested when they knew it would not result in successful treatment. At about the same time that HAART treatment became widely available in Botswana, President Mogae initiated a new "opt-out" program designed to encourage more citizens to get tested to learn their HIV status. Although voluntary testing and counseling centers had existed in Botswana for some time, only a small fraction of the population knew their

HIV status. After the opt-out program began, all those who came to a health facility for any reason were told that routine HIV testing would be done, but that they had the right to refuse it—to opt out. Most people did get tested, and as a result, almost half of Botswana's citizens learned whether they were infected. For those who were infected, this led to a CD4 test and greater assurance that they would receive HAART treatment as soon as they needed such treatment.

It has long been assumed that knowing one's status with respect to HIV would lead to less risky behavior. Those who knew they were HIV positive would presumably want to avoid infecting others (although clearly this is not always the case). However, it could also be argued that the availability of life-saving HAART treatment might lead to riskier sexual behavior, since the individual knows that HIV infection does not necessarily mean near-certain death, as it did in the era of Mma Monica. In California, for example, some have argued that the widespread availability of life-saving HAART has led to an increase in risky, unprotected sex among a new generation of homosexual men.

Uganda is often cited as an example of a country where the epidemic of HIV/AIDS was controlled, with infection rates dropping to about 5 percent from an earlier level of 10 to 15 percent. The epidemic in Uganda and East Africa peaked about a decade before the epidemic in Botswana and the rest of southern Africa. Thus, a very large fraction of the individuals infected as the earlier epidemic expanded died in the 1980s and 1990s, before treatment was available. It is arguable that the high death rate in Uganda resulted in lower rates of new infections. Death by lung cancer in a cigarette-smoking parent is believed to be a strong deterrent to smoking for parent's teenage children. By analogy, we might speculate that widespread deaths from HIV in the era before HAART might reduce rates of infection through risky sex in younger members of the victims' families.

In 1997 in Botswana, AIDS was often called the "new disease," the "radio disease" (that is, the disease people had been hearing about on the radio), or the "disease with no cure." This was obviously before most people were aware that successful HAART treatment was already available in the rich countries. Patients were more likely to consult traditional healers or faith healers, because the local hospitals offered nothing better. Mma Monica died a gruesome death just a few years before she might have been saved with HAART.

· 6 ·

Naledi and Her Nephew Shima

AIDS in Children

NALEDI IS GOOD AT HER JOB, but she does not believe in herself enough and she is always complaining that other staff members are ganging up against her. During lunch breaks, she generally keeps to herself, reading religious materials and surfing the Internet for more spiritual inspiration. She has come to me on many occasions about one slight or another—some of them I daresay imagined—directed at her by some colleague. When she knocked hesitantly on my door one lunch hour in 2003, I assumed that it would be yet another complaint about a coworker who had unfairly blamed her for a missing file or had said unmentionable nasty things behind her back. It was not.

"Judge, I just got a call from Phikwe; from my nephew's teacher. She says something must be done. She says if you see my nephew, you would cry. Yes, ma'am she says it makes a person cry." Naledi was leaning in a bit with her face slightly turned to her left, so that her right ear, not her face, was toward me. Not for the first time, I wondered whether she was a little deaf in her left ear. Or perhaps the turning away was just part of her shy nature. Her eyes had started to redden and tear up. She sniffled and dried her eyes with a corner of her jacket. I knew that Naledi's sister had died of AIDS, leaving a ten-year-old son. I also knew that the father had left the child with his own mother and taken up with a new woman.

"What's the matter? Is the boy ill?"

"The teacher says he comes to school unbathed and hungry. That he looks like a street child. I must go up and see him. Judge, can you talk to them downstairs? I want to leave today. Now! You know how it is; just because it is me, they will come up with all sorts of barriers. No one likes me downstairs. I don't know what my sin is." "Downstairs" is the administration section of the High Court.

"I am sure you can fill in an emergency leave form and get time off for two days or so. I will talk to them."

"Thank you, Judge. You know it breaks my heart that my sister's child should suffer like this when I am alive. I want to take care of him because I love him and because he is used to me and my children. But his grandmother has taken him because it is her duty. She can't look after a ten-year-old child. A sick one too!"

"Why don't you go up? Talk to her and the teachers and see what you can work out. Call me when you get there."

Within an hour, Naledi had left for Phikwe, about 500 kilometers from Lobatse.

"Judge, I am at my nephew's school. You should see this boy. No one is taking care of him. He is dirty and you should see his teeth! You would cry if you were to see him."

"Have you spoken to his grandmother?"

"No, I spent the night with a friend and came to the school directly."

"What do you plan to do?"

"He started crying when he saw me. I have not seen him since the funeral. He grabbed my skirt and would not let me go. He wants to come with me. What am I going to do?"

"First go and talk to the grandmother. Maybe she will be happy to let you take the boy."

"No she won't. She and my father had bad words at the funeral. My father accused her son of killing his daughter. So you see, she will not want to see me."

"Still, go and see her. You never know. She doesn't really know her own grandson and clearly she is not coping with taking care of him. Go and see her first."

"Maybe I should go to the social workers. May be they can recommend that I take the boy with me. I can't leave him. You should see him. He is light in complexion, my own coloring. But you would never guess that. He is dark and streaked with grime. You would cry if you saw him! Really, you would just cry!"

"Where is the father of this child?"

"He is living with another woman down south. He does not take care of him. I understand he is planning to remarry."

Later the same day, Naledi called to report that the grandmother was angry that Naledi had come up to Phikwe without first calling her or otherwise making arrangements with her.

"Do you think she really wants to take care of the child? Or does she feel it is her traditional duty to do so? Maybe she is just embarrassed to let you take the child. She is concerned that people will say she was not able to take care of her grandson."

"I am sure she does not want to take care of the child. She is complaining that it is a lot of work and that people do not appreciate what she is doing."

"I guess, though, that she cannot just hand over the child to you. It would be a traditional sin, almost. So perhaps you can take the child in a way that does not cause her to lose face."

"How?"

"But first, do you really think you are ready to take on another child? You have three boys of your own. Your father is fighting with that woman. You have a sick brother who is insisting his own child be brought into your family." I could just imagine the complications that were likely to result from Naledi's unilateral decision to take in her nephew. She was an unmarried mother of three boys, and bringing in a fourth was bound to create ripples within her own nuclear family. In addition, although her decision was to take the child to her own home, because she was unmarried, it would be understood that she was taking the child on behalf of her parents and birth family. The other family, the boy's father's family, had given *bogadi*, or *lobola* (marriage payment, usually in cattle), for Naledi's sister, so the child belonged to them. Naledi, a mere sister of the deceased, could not, without the mandate of her father, just walk into the schoolyard and take away the child. Such a mandate would ordinarily be given after a family meeting, at which all the family members would give their views.

"Judge, I can't leave him. I will just have to see that I cope, somehow!"

"What will your father say?"

"I don't know. My brother will be angry, though. He says why should we take care of a child whose father is alive and who has given *bogadi*. His own girlfriend died, leaving a child, and he wants to force us to take in the child."

Naledi came from a family plagued by infighting; fists had been known to fly among the brothers, and she had on occasion had to barricade herself in her room at her parents' house when one of her brothers had flown into one of his legendary tempers. Naledi lives in her own house in Lobatse, but taking her nephew in would mean that the child would be part of her family, visiting her parents' family on weekends and school holidays. The brother's views could not simply be ignored.

"Where is the boy right now?"

"He is holding on to my dress. He will not let me go. He is begging me not to leave him."

"Okay. Here is my suggestion. At this point, the natural guardian of that child is his father. He has left him under the care of his own mother, who is, if what you say is correct, not coping. Sit down and compose a letter to the school and the local social worker, explaining why you came to Phikwe, that you must return to work, and that you are unable to leave the child in the condition that he is in. Explain that you are taking him with you to Lobatse, where you work, and that you would be happy for an assessment of who is best suited to get custody of the boy. Explain that you are taking him with you only because you believe it would be irresponsible to leave him behind. Describe his condition in full; that is, his state of dress, hygiene, and health. Then get on a bus with that boy and deal with the consequences."

The following day Naledi came into my office, and attached to her dress was a dazed little boy who indeed could easily cause one to dissolve into tears. His lips were a mess of sores and his gums were bleeding. His eyes were watery—whether with tears or an infection, it was not clear; perhaps a mixture of both.

"Judge, you can see that I could not leave him behind? My sister cannot rest in peace if we do this to her child."

"*Dumela papa,*" I addressed the boy. He stiffened and whispered a hello back.

"How old are you?"

"He is ten, but he looks six! I just can't believe that someone can do this to a child. Not washing him, not feeding him. Judge, he was crying in the bus yesterday."

Naledi explained that she had come to work not only so I could see the child for myself, but also so she could request more time off to take him to the hospital.

Over the next months, Naledi shared with me the developments in her nephew's life. She reported to me that the boy's father, who had remarried, had succumbed to AIDS, and that suddenly the grandmother, who had not lifted a finger when the child was taken from her, wanted custody. The boy's parents had both been civil servants, meaning that there was money due to their son and that the parents had taken out life insurance policies; whoever took the boy would get control of the money. This pot of money was behind a year-long legal custody battle, during which unkind words were flung back and forth.

As the custody case continued, Naledi started to be worried about the health of the boy. That he could have been infected was a very great possibility. Both his parents had died of AIDS, and he was sickly. Just as one sore disappeared another erupted, and his lymph nodes were perpetually swollen

"Judge, I am thinking of having Shima tested for HIV."

"Do you think you are ready for the results? How is the counseling going?"

"Oh, Judge, I don't know what I would do without the counseling. Life is hard, Judge. Life has been hard!"

"How are your children reacting to Shima? His living with you?"

"Life is hard, Judge. At home and at work."

"Are you sure they are not jealous? This past year you have concentrated on Shima, and if you are not careful, they will begin to be resentful." I had observed Naledi put a lot of passion and time into problems associated with bringing her nephew into her house. Even as the custody case raged on, she fought for and succeeded in having some of the boy's money released to her so she could enroll him in a private school, put him on a good balanced diet, and ensure that he received good medical attention. She would take a day off at short notice if the boy required anything at all.

"Oh, you are right! Of course you are right. My oldest son is being difficult! The counselor says he is jealous. He refuses counseling though. He says he is not mad. You see, Shima goes to private school while they do not. Shima's problems have consumed us this past year; the legal battle, his hospital visits, the fights . . . But what can I do? I just couldn't let him die in Phikwe!"

"Have you told your own children all of this?"

"I tell them that he is ill and his mother died; so they should have sympathy."

"Yes, but they still want their mother. They probably feel neglected. About the testing, I have spoken to Dr. Rebecca Tucker. She will see you and give advice."

"Hi, Unity, this is Rebecca. You sent someone over to see me. Naledi? She has a nephew whose parents died of AIDS."

"Yes. She is considering having the child tested."

"I understand there is a custody case going, so she may, if she loses the case, lose the boy."

"Yes, that is a possibility."

"Well, my suggestion is that we wait for the court decision. The child is doing well right now as it is. I can treat the infections. It would be best if the real guardian is the one who has the child tested and then embarks on a long-term treatment plan.

"I also think that Naledi should continue with counseling. She appears to be overwhelmed. Being a single mother of four boys, fighting a legal case, and worrying that your nephew is HIV positive is a lot for one person."

"I hear you. Thank you."

"I will continue to see the boy and will not hesitate to have him tested if I think his health condition calls for that. In the meantime, I do not think that there is any urgency to test him. It will not necessarily help him right now."

The day did come when the testing could not wait any longer. The child was plagued by opportunistic infections, especially flu and what seemed to be herpes. His mouth was a mess of sores, rotten teeth, and persistently bleeding gums.

"Judge, he is positive. I know this should not be a surprise, but couldn't God have spared him? His parents are dead. Wasn't that enough?"

"How did Shima take it?"

"He cried and cried when he was told."

"What does Dr. Magawa say?" Naledi had just come back from the pediatrics branch of the Princess Marina Hospital.

"He says he will be fine. But you know doctors—always saying patients will be fine!"

"When does he start on his HIV drugs?"

"Not yet. They still have to check his CD4 cell count and his viral load. We have to go back next week and I don't know how many more times before he starts. But the people there are really nice. I just hope their medicines work. But they really are nice and patient."

"Judge, I won the custody case! That is such a relief. I could not sleep, just thinking Shima would go back to Phikwe. It would have killed me. And him.

"Judge, I want to thank you and Judge Dibeela. I remember what he said after the two of you had talked. He said to me, 'Mma, these days there is medication that can help; people are tested and put on medication and they go on with their lives. I am not saying this child of your sister is ill [with AIDS] but he might be one of the unfortunate ones; just go and test him and if he is sick put him on treatment, he will be okay.' It was those words that gave me the courage to have Shima tested."

Shima has been put on a drug trial to see which drugs work best.

Naledi's boys continue to fight, and recently the tension has caused Naledi to go back to counseling. The eldest continues to refuse counseling, which takes place at the Lobatse Mental Hospital, insisting that he is not mad.

About the two-year-long ordeal, Naledi says, "Every time I think of this, a tear falls. I don't understand whether it is a tear of joy or a tear of pity."

Naledi's sister died of AIDS, leaving a ten-year-old son who was apparently not being properly cared for. The boy, Shima, was left with his paternal grandmother. Shima's father also died of AIDS some time later, after marrying another woman. Shima was eventually diagnosed with HIV/AIDS and put on antiretroviral therapy.

The timing of the HIV infections illustrates the prolonged and variable window that exists between initial infection and disease development. Regardless of accusations by Naledi's father that her sister's husband killed her sister by infecting her with HIV, it is impossible to know at that point whether the mother of the boy infected the father, or the father infected the mother. It is even possible, though unlikely, that each parent became infected by someone else. Either way, the now-deceased mother must have infected Shima around the time of birth or breastfeeding.

In some instances it may be possible to tell who infected an adult, but only if a blood sample is checked within a few months of the new infection and a sample is also available from the potential donor partner or partners. This is done by performing a test called a gene sequence analysis, in which the letters in the genetic code of the virus are examined for identity or similarity between the potential donor and the recipient. This works only with recent infections; after several years the accumulation of mutations clouds the analysis. Because Shima's mother and father were presumably both infected six to ten years before they were diagnosed, it would be too late at this point to track the source of the infection.

Apart from the unusual situation of a transfusion with contaminated blood, there is really no way for a child to become infected between the ages of about two and twelve. Breastfeeding would presumably end by age two or three at the latest, and risk of sexual exposure should not arise until puberty, at age twelve to fourteen. Early in the epidemic, when it was already known that HIV could be transmitted by sex or blood transfusions, some wondered whether HIV could also be transmitted by mosquitoes who suck infected blood, as with malaria. It was soon apparent that HIV was not transmitted by mosquitoes, because children from ages three to ten often have the greatest number of mosquito bites but do not develop new cases of HIV infection.

Some children infected by their mothers show evidence of disease within the first year or two, and die soon after. These are most likely to be children who were infected before birth, even before their immune systems were fully formed. While infants infected by breastfeeding may be a bit more susceptible when they first begin to take the milk, it is clear that breastfeeding infections can occur as long as the child is still getting milk from an HIV-positive mother, at least until they are two years old. Children who get infected later, such as at two years of age, may have a longer induction period before developing clinical AIDS. We could speculate that this is what happened to Shima, as he apparently did not show signs of AIDS disease until he was seven or eight. However, individual differences in the time taken to develop disease may also be related to genetic variation. This includes both genetic variation between HIVs, some of which cause disease more rapidly, and genetic differences between people, some of whom show better immune protection from progression.

Children with AIDS have many of the same signs and symptoms seen in adults: persistent diarrhea, low-grade fever, respiratory problems, swollen lymph glands, and mouth infections due to yeast or herpes. The chronic sores that Shima had around the teeth and lips were probably due to the herpesvirus. When the yeast is growing it may appear white, and the infected area usually smells. Shima also had persistent lymphadenopathy, a condition of generalized swollen lymph glands that often precedes full-blown AIDS in both children and adults.

Most of the drugs used to prevent or treat opportunistic infections in adults can be used in children, but are given in lower doses according to the weight of the child. Children who are infected with HIV have higher rates of disease and death from a wide variety of illnesses, as compared to children who are not infected with HIV. However, children who are born to HIV-infected mothers but remain uninfected still have higher rates of disease and death when compared with uninfected children born to uninfected mothers. This may be because the children do not get as much immune protection from their mothers' milk, or because an ill mother is less able to provide care to the child.

The antiretroviral drugs used to attack HIV in children are also the same as the drugs used to treat adults. However, much less information is available about which drugs work best, how best to avoid toxicities, and how to diminish the development and persistence of drug resistance in children. Most of the detailed research trials that compare such drugs for safety and efficacy have been done in the United States or Europe. And because most HIV-infected people in the developed countries are injection-drug users or homosexual men, much less is known about how drug effects or benefits may be different in women or children. In the United States, only about a hundred infants are newly infected each year; even if all participated in research trials, the numbers are often too small to yield statistically valid information. In some areas of southern Africa, up to a tenth of all children may get infected, but the infrastructure, medical expertise, and financial resources needed to conduct clinical treatment trials are usually not available. Thus the medical treatment of children with AIDS is less than ideal. Despite this, treatment is usually successful, and children who are treated can lead successful lives.

Diagnosis of the initial HIV infection is also more difficult in young children. When a child is older than eighteen to twenty months, HIV can be diagnosed with simple antibody tests, as it is in adults. However, children younger than that still have antibodies they received from their mother, including HIV antibodies. Although they don't seem to offer any protection against infection, these antibodies should not be taken as an indicator of the presence of HIV in the child. All children born to HIV-infected mothers have such antibodies, whether they are infected or not. To verify that the infant is not infected, a polymerase chain reaction test must be performed, using a few drops of the infant's blood. This test, if positive, directly detects the virus, avoiding the possibility of a false-positive test, which often occurs with antibody tests in young children.

The guilty feelings that Naledi has concerning the care of Shima also illustrate the familial ties that are typical of extended families in Botswana. Aunts and grandmothers are expected to take care of grandchildren or the children of siblings—even when they require very extensive care, such as that needed by an AIDS patient. It has been estimated that there are currently about 15 million orphans in the world who became orphans because of HIV/AIDS. The vast majority are in sub-Saharan Africa. A large fraction of the children in Botswana have lost one or both parents to AIDS.

It Is the Will of God

HIV and Tuberculosis

WHEN TIMID THABO literally accosted me in the corridor leading to my office, I assumed that he was still angry with me for my
daring to suggest that his Bible reading and weekend preaching
were not enough to deal with his declining health. After weeks
of my trying, unsuccessfully, to get him to accept that he was ill,
he had unceremoniously dumped me for another judge who lived
within five minutes of the courthouse. Then rumors started to fly
around the office that I had demanded a change of drivers because I
claimed that Thabo had TB. His coughing, it was said, was really the
result of his having to drive long distances to pick me up, of the
dusty patch of road leading off from the tar-paved road to my house,
and my unreasonable preference for air conditioning at rather low
temperatures. I was an insensitive and unfair boss, was the general
sentiment. Nothing was said of the financial benefits of driving others, outside the work hours, which had originally attracted Thabo to
driving me in the first place, an incentive that generated a clutch of
drivers begging to replace him. My attempts to get Thabo to sit
down for a talk about the matter had been met with excuses on his
part. I thought he would never talk to me again.

"Judge, I want to tell you that I did go to the hospital. You were right, I have TB, but I am on treatment now. That is all I had, TB, and I am being treated. I have to go to the hospital every morning, so you see, I cannot drive an out-of-Lobatse judge. But I am going to be okay. I placed my health in the hands of the Lord, and I am going to be okay."

"That's great. Come to my office. Let's talk a bit more."

"I have to go, Judge. I have to take my judge to Gabs now. He is waiting for me."

A step had been taken, and though clearly not enough, it was something. He still had not tested for HIV, but at least he was talking to me again.

Thabo is a slow, soft-spoken person. Until you put him behind a steering wheel, and then he turns into a careful but sure-footed and confident individual. He was arguably the best driver I had been assigned in the eight years I had worked as a judge, and I had come to trust his ability to negotiate the rather dangerous eighty or so kilometers from the office to my house. He was deeply religious and it seemed he worried about my soul, for he would leave religious materials on my seat, in my briefcase, and sometimes on my table. I knew that he was a preacher of sorts, but I had never heard him preach. Those who had claimed that Thabo, cloaked in the blue and white robes of his church, was transformed into a preacher whose voice and bearing bore no relationship to those of the timid, low-paid driver known to me.

Even though I never read the literature he left for me, out of politeness I made it a point to move the materials so he would not think I was ignoring his gestures. He was not a big talker and I preferred to read during our trips back and forth between the court and my home, so our relationship was cordial but not familiar. For example, when he had gotten married a few years previously, I had bought him a present, even though I did not attend the wedding, and when his first child was born, he had informed me of the fact and I had congratulated him.

The breakdown in our relationship had started when first his breath started to smell really bad, and then his chest started to be racked with coughs, suggesting to me that he was not well.

"Judge, is there a difference between the spirit and the soul?" The question interrupted a bout of coughing, and I wondered whether it was actually timed to do just that. Thabo had been coughing for months and the frequency was increasing. And although he had never been a big man, he seemed to be losing weight as well.

"I can't say I have given it much thought, actually. And, I don't want to seem like I am harassing you, but you really must see a doctor about that cough."

"It's the dust on this road, Judge." There was terseness in his voice. Thabo's practice of leaving Scripture verses and other religious materials on my seat seemed to have escalated, so that there was no longer any surreptitiousness about it. It seemed to me that since the onset of AIDS and death had become ever-present occurrences, preachers were erupting everywhere, and the High Court was no different. The last time we had discussed his coughing, brought on by carrying my briefcase up a short flight of stairs, a Bible had tumbled out of his pocket and landed at my feet. The repeated message was clear: all was in the hands of the Lord, and heathen me, I was meddling in matters way above my head.

I had seen enough HIV-infected people to suspect that Thabo might indeed be infected with the virus. My concern was that every day that went by without his being tested, and therefore without being treated, was going to make it that much harder to reverse the ravages of opportunistic illnesses associated with AIDS. Every day that went by also exposed his wife and young children to the possibility of TB infection. And I also had personal concerns. Thabo and I were spending, on average, 130 minutes every day, Monday to Friday, together in a small, air-conditioned sedan, and his coughing was a cause of concern for myself as well. TB is highly infectious, and every time his slight frame was racked by a bout of coughing I could almost see the germs flying my way. As a young child, before TB was nearly eradicated from the population, I had seen two cousins die of the disease and a niece become waiflike before finally returning to good health, and only after months of treatment and special feeding.

The coughing had been preceded by weeks of the rather bad mouth odor, the probable reasons for which I had first raised with him in a note that I had written for him to read later, in the privacy of the car.

"Thabo, don't take this the wrong way, but have you ever heard of gum disease?" I had then explained to him what that was and that since he had always had very good oral hygiene, his bad breath could have other sources than merely failing to brush his teeth. I told him that the care with which he was moving his mouth suggested to me that he had mouth sores. Thabo had been understandably embarrassed by my raising the issue, but I had long decided that too many lives had been lost while politeness had been allowed to rank higher than common sense.

"I am sorry that I did not brush my teeth this morning. Maybe it was what I ate."

My response was gentle but firm, "No, Thabo, this is not about your not brushing your teeth well enough. This is about your possibly—I am not saying definitely, but possibly—having some kind of infection in your mouth. There could be many reasons. Only a doctor can tell you the reasons." I then told him the story of a close member of my family, how he developed mouth sores that he ignored, how his breath started to smell, and how he did not go to see the doctor until he started having diarrhea and could no longer deny that he was very ill.

"He has been on ARVs now for a year, and he is doing very well.

But we nearly lost him. I am sure you know of similar stories . . ." I could see that Thabo did not want to listen to me. His face was set in a tight mask and only the official relationship between us stopped him from telling me to shut up and mind my own business.

"Thabo, please think about what I have just said. Talk to someone you trust."

"Yes, Judge. Can I go now? I need to go and put in petrol. What time are we leaving today?" I had no choice but to get out of the vehicle and to let him drive off to the petrol station.

After numerous similar discussions, Thabo had decided that he did not want to work with me anymore.

As his reputation as a preacher grew, he became one of the preferred staff members to lead the morning HIV/AIDS prayer sessions at the court. Over months, he put his energy into praying for others, deflecting attention from his own health.

Finally he could not deny his own illness any more; the coughing must have become too much to bear, and reluctantly he had gone to the hospital. When he was told he had TB, he had decided to wave this explanation at everyone who asked after his health, hoping to use it as a shield against any further questions.

"I have TB, not AIDS," he seemed to want to shout to all who would listen.

❖

Thabo is a deeply religious man who was initially reluctant to accept that he is ill. While he finally gets a diagnosis of TB and admits that to others, he is even more reluctant to get tested for HIV. It is likely that he did get tested for HIV when he received the TB diagnosis but doesn't want to admit it. Most physicians would feel compelled to test for HIV and immune functions when TB occurs in a region with a high prevalence of HIV, such as Botswana. Thabo's mouth sores and bad breath are also associated with thrush and other oral lesions, such as hairy leukoplakia, that often occur in AIDS patients, including those who don't have TB. So there would be an immediate suspicion that he had more than just TB. Additionally, some of the drugs used to treat TB can interact with certain medications used to treat HIV/AIDS, so the treating physician or nurse would have several reasons to want to know Thabo's HIV status.

A very large fraction of the people of Africa are infected with the bacterium that causes TB, *Mycobacterium tuberculosis*. Even before the HIV epidemic existed in the human population, TB infected a large number of people, especially those who were poor and living under crowded conditions with poor sanitation. However, more than 90 percent of the people who become infected with this bacterium don't get the disease. The disease occurs primarily when the body is weakened by something else. That something else could be poor nutrition, or cancer. But that something else is now overwhelmingly HIV, at least in Africa. At present, at least three-fourths of the people who have active TB disease in southern Africa have it because of HIV. They have the severe coughing and the clouded lungs that appear on X-ray pictures of the chest. Those who are infected with TB but not with HIV are much more likely to control the infection, so that a few bacteria smolder in latent form but cause no real disease. Those who are also infected with HIV are more likely to get more severe cases of TB. While it is usually limited to the lungs, in HIV-infected people TB is more likely to spread to other places as well, such as the bones or the surfaces of the heart or brain.

Unlike HIV, TB is spread by air-borne bacteria, through coughing, spitting, and sneezing. This is a major reason why public health rules were directed against spitting in public places, and why physicians and nurses wash their hands between patients. If a TB patient coughs or sneezes into his hand and then shakes the hand of another person, this can readily transmit TB. So the judge was indeed justified in her concerns that the hacking coughs of Thabo, especially while driving in the car, could pose a risk for others in the same space, including herself. Thabo also exposed his wife and children to TB, whether or not they were infected with HIV.

TB disease occurs primarily in very poor countries or regions, and among poor populations, whether or not it is associated with HIV. In the United States, for example, TB rates are highest in the homeless population, in that small proportion of people who are very poor or mentally ill, and have not been helped by the social structure. In Africa and Asia prior to the epidemic of HIV, TB was already a big problem in the poorest countries. Since AIDS, it has become much worse. Botswana, Namibia, and South Africa are the richest countries in Africa on a per capita basis. However, even in these countries up to half of the people are very poor. Prior to the economic progress of the past thirty years in Botswana, TB was a major problem. Now, it has become an even greater problem because of the HIV epidemic.

Within recent years, the epidemic of TB in southern Africa has also become a huge problem because an increasing proportion of patients are infected with drug-resistant strains. The multidrug-resistant (MDR) strains of TB are resistant to both of the drugs that are usually used for TB treatment. Other multidrug-resistant TB bacteria may be labeled XTB, or extremely resistant TB, when the disease does not respond to any of the drugs that are generally available. This is another way that the HIV epidemic is making the TB epidemic even worse. Along with the increase in rates of TB, the fraction of TB cases that are MDR is also increasing.

After Thabo announced that he had TB, he stated that he had to go to the hospital every morning for treatment, so he could not drive for Judge Dow. Whether he is being treated for HIV or TB, it would seem unlikely that he'd have to go to the hospital every day for the treatment. A program called directly observed therapy, or

DOT, is often followed for TB, and sometimes for HIV. In this program, the patient must be observed taking the drugs to avoid lapses, as interruptions in taking the drugs cause drug resistance. However, the person doing the DOT observations usually is not a physician or nurse at a hospital. It is usually a family member or friend who is selected by the patient. It is remotely possible, but un-likely, that the person designated to give Thabo his drugs for TB is based at the hospital. If so, he would have to go to that site so the observer could verify that he took the drugs.

Thabo also seems to hide behind his religion to avoid the reality that he needs to verify his HIV status, which in his case seems psy-chologically as well as medically confounded by the TB. A few years ago in Africa, learning that one was infected with HIV might have been interpreted as a death sentence. But this is no longer true in Botswana for those who can accept their diagnosis and adhere to the drug schedule for therapy. Let's hope that Thabo sees the light of modern medicine, not just the light of his religion.

Walking Skeletons and Hesitant Hugs

Toxicities and Resistance to Drugs Used to Treat HIV/AIDS

RANKO WAS SIXTEEN YEARS OLD when his maternal grandfather made a decision that saved his life but nixed his chance of a high school education. Ranko's brother had died after being bewitched by an uncle intent on taking over the boys' herd of cattle. The boys had just buried their own father when their uncle, whom they had never met, because he had long before deserted the extended family to work in the mines in South Africa, returned. The uncle claimed the boys' herd of cattle and when the boys challenged him, he decided to kill them through witchcraft. Ranko's brother's death was easy to engineer, for he allowed his uncle to *phekola* (cure) him, thus allowing his uncle direct contact with his body; a few ritual cuts, deadly medicine rubbed into the bleeding wounds, and before long, the boy was dead. Ranko was smart enough to see the danger, so he refused to submit. The uncle found other indirect ways to attack him, and Ranko was soon plagued by mysterious spells that would freeze him in one spot, rendering him mute for hours. When one traditional doctor after another diagnosed the diabolic doings of the uncle, Ranko's maternal grandfather saw no other option but to take the frail boy into his care. He removed him from his paternal village and kept him at his cattle post, away from the clutches of the murderous and thieving uncle.

"Let the boy come stay with me so he can remain in school," a paternal aunt entreated.

"What is the use of education if the boy ends up dead?" the grandfather reasoned.

For Ranko's mother, who was then a widow, sending her only child off to live with her own parents would have been a very hard decision to make. It would have been seen as a comment on the health of her relationship with her husband's family. The young widow stood firm, though; it was better to have a son you hardly saw than one who was dead.

The spells were finally cured by a particularly good traditional doctor, but the uncle still had his eye on the boys' cattle and did not give up trying to kill the boy. The only sure way to save Ranko was to raise him with his mother's people, and that is where he remained until he was old enough to make his own way in the world.

Since his maternal grandfather lived at his cattle post, away from the village, that meant Ranko had to stop going to school. Five years passed before it was deemed safe to allow the boy to move back to the village, and by that time any chance of going to high school had long passed. By that time, too, his uncle had dispossessed Ranko of his inheritance, so the young man had to go penniless into the world to make his living.

Ranko had been working as an unskilled laborer for two years when he was diagnosed with TB. This was in 1979. He was hospitalized, and for sixty days, every morning without fail, a nurse jabbed his backside with an injection of medication. After some time, when he lay on his bed he could spread his legs only with difficulty, his backside was so sore. Then he started to lose his sight and it was determined that he had been overdosed. His sight has since remained impaired.

"I survived an uncle intent on killing me and then a medicine that nearly blinded me! I thought I had received my share of bad things, and then in 1989 I had the most curious illness! From nowhere, I would be seized with searing heat. All over my body, I would feel hot and pour down with sweat. For days this went on. It was like I had malaria. But at the hospital, they said I did not have malaria. But my body told me I was not fine. I don't know how to explain it. My whole body felt like there was . . . it was like something was boiling inside. It would come and go and I was sure something strange was going on inside me. After a while, I was fine and I forgot about it. But even today, when I remember that feeling . . . I am sure that is when my body was fighting the virus."

In 1999 Ranko started to get ill again.

"My sister, I was coughing," he told me. "Coughing and coughing! You heard me coughing, you were sure that I was about to die."

A private doctor diagnosed Ranko as having AIDS. He was put on ARVs.

"Within a month you could not believe it was me. I had stopped coughing, and I had gained back my weight. These pills work like magic, I tell you. Those days you really had to hide the fact that you were infected . . . You did not tell anyone . . . Those were lonely years . . ."

Those were the years of walking skeletons and hesitant hugs. Visitors were known to sit upwind from a sick person, just on the off chance that the deadly virus might blow their way. Cups were scrubbed and carefully rinsed after being used by an infected person. Gloves were recommended during the bathing of patients. They were years of whispers and fear. Ranko was relieved to be back on his feet, and no doubt, with witchcraft all around, his collapse and amazing recovery would always be explained in those terms.

Within one year though, Ranko had exhausted his limit under his medical insurance and the plan would not pay for his drugs any longer. He could not afford to pay for the drugs himself, so he stopped taking them.

"I could not afford to buy the drugs. And, to tell you the truth, I told myself that I had been cured. Even you, if you had seen me, you would not have believed that I still had this illness in my blood. I looked healthy and strong. So, I did not try to find other ways to pay for the drugs. Also, taking drugs was stressful. . . . Always hiding them . . . always afraid someone will find them."

One year later, though, Ranko was near death once again.

"I heard over the radio that you must not stop taking the drugs; that you will get ill again. I knew then that the illness had returned."

Since he could not afford private health care, Ranko went to a government clinic. He pretended that he did not know his status, so he was retested. His wife was tested as well, and she too was found to be positive.

"Oh, I tell you, my sister, those early years! There was so much fear. I thought everyone will reject me, like a diseased dog! I had survived so much and now I was sick with an embarrassing disease. Even the doctors and the nurses—you were afraid to tell them the truth. When they gave me the drugs, I realized that they were exactly what I had taken before. I was sure I was going to be fine."

Ranko was determined to take his drugs as directed by the doctor; he would not miss a dose. He and his wife took their drugs at the same time, and if he was not home, he would call his wife to remind her that it was time to take her medication. He even set alarm reminders on his cell phone. He was determined that he would take his drugs every day and at exactly the recommended time.

"But the drugs did not work. They had to change them. I was taking them exactly as the doctors had said and they did not work. They were exactly the same drugs that had worked so well two years before!"

Ranko is a very intelligent man and he has acquired useful skills during the various jobs he has held, so that even with only a primary-school education he has made a fairly successful life for himself and his family, which comprises his wife and three children, two of whom were born to his wife before the pair married. He is proud that they own their own house while some families are renters. He worries about his children, growing up during these days of HIV/AIDS.

Ranko believes that his wife was infected around the time that he was very ill in 1999. This was a year after they married and the year of the birth of their third child. The child has since tested negative, much to the relief of the parents.

Ranko recalls the secrecy with which he used to take his drugs. His cell phone alarm would go off, and if he was in the company of friends or colleagues he would look at it, pretending it was a text message coming in. He would mutter something, pretending that it was in response to the message. He would then allow a few minutes to go by and excuse himself to go to the toilet. In the privacy of a toilet stall, he would carefully take out his pills, pop them into his mouth, and emerge to the more public part of the toilet to surreptitiously swallow them with handfuls of water. For years, he and his wife took their drugs without the knowledge of any of their children. Recently they told their eldest child, but the two youngest, ages sixteen and eleven, have not been told.

"Oh! Now taking drugs comes as naturally as wearing a seat belt. No one has to remind me. I don't have to remind my wife. It's what we do every day as directed. We never forget. And recently they changed my drugs again, but this time they say one of them is actually two drugs."

The drugs worked fine for Ranko's wife, and she remains on that first set of drugs prescribed for her in 2003. The drugs, though, did not work for at least two of Ranko's acquaintances, two women with whom he shared the then long lines at the health clinic, before the system started to cope with the demands made on it.

One of those women was Sarah K. Sarah's CD4 cell count was five when she was first put on ARV drugs. On her first visit to the clinic she sat bent and gaunt on the bench, not joining in the chatter of those around her—her mind was on her three children back home. She was thirty-nine, unmarried. She had also seen lots of people dying of AIDS.

Over time though, the waiting room became a place to see friends and trade hopeful stories. People you had seen literally carried in sometime before would be glowing, and discussing the future with confidence. It was with a heart full of hope that Sarah took home her first set of pills, but that hope was dashed when she was told that the drugs were not taming her raging viral load. She was put on a second set of drugs, but the drugs made her ill, something to do with her pancreas. The next set of drugs did not work either, and as if she did not have enough problems, she was diagnosed with cervical cancer. She is now on her fourth set of drugs. She puts forward a brave face, but occasionally she simply falls apart with hopelessness.

Tlotlo, the other woman for whom the drugs did not work, is on her fourth set of drugs as well. She is twenty-eight years old and was twenty-four when she first went on ARV drugs.

"The man who infected me died in 2006. I was in a bus and I overheard someone saying that he was ill and in the hospital. You know how men are, when you get ill they leave you . . . I called him and he sounded so ill. He died the following day . . . I was a naive girl. I had thought he loved me. Then when I was ill, he did not want to know me . . . That is how Gaborone men are. I am at peace with it all now."

Tlotlo has been recently diagnosed with TB and she blames her work environment for that; colleagues who have TB are allowed to continue to work in the closed factory environment, reusing the same masks and aprons for five days at a time. She has taken unpaid leave from her ninety-dollars-per-month job so that she can receive TB treatment. Tlotlo lives with her parents and two sisters, each of whom has a young child. She has never earned enough to leave home, and with only three years of high school education her prospects are limited. She worries about her two sisters, especially the youngest one.

"I have stopped worrying about myself. I am at peace with my condition now, although I am a bit angry about this TB thing. I was doing fine . . . I am worried about my sister . . . really worried. She must look at me and see where she is headed if she does not listen to our counsel."

Tlotlo says her sister is having an affair with a man who processes scholarship applications at the Ministry of Education. Through his work he meets young girls hoping for scholarships, and every year he gets a new girlfriend.

"My sister thinks this man has power. He is just one of many clerks! He is just using her. But she does not listen. My mother has given up. Three people on drugs in my family; my parents and I! Now I have TB. I am unemployed. My two sisters have young children! I will never have a child. I don't want a man, either. I tell you, when they first told me that my drugs were not working I just thought, 'Whatever God decides.' Now I am on my fourth set of drugs, but the last one was because of what they say is National something—Truvada, ALU and RIT, something like that—ask the nurses . . . I am not sure why they changed . . . Am I talking too much? I am really worried about my sisters and my TB. Some people say I must look for a boyfriend with HIV, and, yes . . . I have seen people meet on those long lines and later get married . . . but even a man with HIV can leave you . . . men just leave you when they see another woman . . . You know, I am really worried about my sister . . . She says I am jealous of her . . . I know in my heart that by the time she comes back to her senses, she will be infected. She does not take care of her child . . . she just thinks of her boyfriend all the time . . . When he calls she leaves whatever she was doing and runs to him . . . Even today . . . we were together and her phone rang and . . . Look at me . . . my ideal weight is fifty-four kilograms but I weigh thirty-five . . . it is this TB. When I first started the TB drugs they made me throw up . . . I hope my HIV drugs will not stop working . . . What future do I have? No husband, no child, and my drugs do not always work. If my sister becomes ill and my parents' drugs do not work . . . But I should not think like that . . . I am at peace . . . really . . . it is my sister I worry about . . . Do I talk too much? Do I worry too much? My parents are on drugs . . . My sister is trying her best to get HIV . . . Three people in one family . . . it is too much."

Ranko, Sarah, and Tlotlo are all AIDS patients being treated with antiretroviral drugs. They are all AIDS patients who have been through several different regimens of drugs. This is not the case for most patients on ARV therapy. All AIDS patients in Botswana's national treatment program begin therapy with the three-drug combination referred to as highly active antiretroviral therapy, or HAART.

Ranko started his drug treatment program before the national ARV treatment program (the Masa program) was begun in late 2001 and early 2002. He was being treated by a private medical practitioner. Initially the drugs worked well and made him "healthy and strong." He stopped taking the drugs because his medical insurance money ran out and he had no way to pay for them. This was a common problem before the national program was in place. It is still a common problem in some other countries in Africa, where AIDS patients are started on drugs and then cannot continue because they have no money.

In some countries, AIDS patients are started on government programs and then turned over to private practitioners, where treatment failure becomes much more likely. The failures occur not only because the patients run out of money; the local physicians and pharmacies may also run out of drugs. Sometimes the patients can get only one or two drugs of the three-drug combination, but it is often more dangerous to take one or two of the drugs than to stop altogether. If the patient takes just one or two, this often accelerates the development of drug resistance. After drug resistance develops, the HIV-1–resistant viruses accumulate in the DNA of the immune cells. They then stay in the body for long periods of time and rapidly emerge if the same drug, or a related drug that has the same drug-resistance profile, is used.

About one in four or five patients who start HAART do not continue with this first line of therapy because of toxic side effects. These toxicities are rarely life threatening, but they may make the patient so sick that he stops taking the drugs. Or he may stop taking one or two of the three, if he thinks he knows which one is causing the diarrhea and vomiting. This, then, leads to the greater problems of drug resistance, just as it does when patients stop taking one or two drugs for reasons of access or cost.

The toxic side effects are often different for particular drugs, or sets of drugs, and are more commonly seen with the least expensive drugs, which are more likely to be available in Africa. The drugs that are less expensive (and sometimes have the greatest toxicity) are more likely to be used by populations that have few financial resources. They may be less expensive because they are no longer covered by patents and generic equivalents may be available, manufactured by companies in the developing world. The large Western pharmaceutical companies that first developed and sold the drugs may also be more willing to "give them up" because they have been largely replaced by newer and better drugs in the United States and Europe. In addition to being less expensive, the drugs produced as generics are also more likely to be available in combinations that work well together in single pills. Western pharmaceutical companies, which are in competition with each other, have less incentive to combine their own products with those from other companies.

The toxic side effects that are commonly seen with ARVs include gastrointestinal problems, such as nausea, vomiting, and diarrhea, as well as anemia and skin rashes, but they can also include peripheral neuropathies, which lead to muscle weakness or numbness and lack of control of the hands and feet. Less common, but more dangerous, are problems with the liver or pancreas, and mitochondrial toxicities or lactic acidosis. These effects are harder to diagnose without laboratory tests and may cause major damage in cells by depriving the cells of their ability to process oxygen. Sarah apparently had a violent reaction to her second-line therapy, which caused pancreatitis. Pancreatitis is often associated with severe abdominal pain as well as nausea and vomiting.

As more and newer drugs were discovered and marketed, techniques for adapting the drugs for slow release and for formulation into a single pill or capsule were also developed. Thus, the medications Combivir, Truvada, Trizivir, and Atripla combine two or three drugs in the same pill. Previously each drug was in a separate pill, and each pill might have had to be taken two or three times each day. With combinations in the same slow-release pill, the patient may have to take only one pill each day. However, like the newer drugs, developments in technology to deliver several drugs together in the same pill, or pills that can be taken less often because they release the drugs slowly, are often not available in Africa until much later.

Greater difficulties in taking the drugs obviously increase the chance that the patient will miss doses. The more missed doses, the higher the chance that drug resistance will develop. Missed doses might also be more likely when the patient is afraid to reveal that he is sick because of the stigma of AIDS. Ranko tells, for example, how he would excuse himself so he could take his drugs in the privacy of a toilet stall. He and his wife also took their drugs without revealing this to their teenage children.

Before drug treatment began to be available in Africa, some Western officials suggested that HAART wouldn't work there because, as they put it, "many people in Africa have never seen a clock or a watch" and "don't know what Western time is." This was, at best, nonsense, as a patient could simply learn to take the pills at sunrise and sunset, or when doing some routine daily activity such as eating or listening to the radio. In fact, the compliance for taking pills on schedule has often been better in Africa than in the United States. In Botswana, a recent study indicated that patients took their drugs on schedule 90 percent of the time. This is surely one of the reasons why the patients there have done so well on HAART. In the national program, the five-year survival rate is 80 percent, even though many patients began taking drugs later, after their immune systems were more damaged, compared with when patients begin on HAART drugs in the developed world. In a research study conducted by the Botswana-Harvard Partnership, 94 percent of the treated patients were alive after two and a half years on therapy. These survival estimates are better than many seen in the best hospitals in the United States and Europe. However, probably a larger percentage of the AIDS patients in developed countries were also alcoholics or intravenous drug abusers, which could have interfered with their ability to take the AIDS drugs. The Botswana study also tested the possible contribution of a *mopati,* a friend or family member who is charged with the responsibility of ensuring that the patient takes his or her drugs on time. This "buddy system" approach was shown to be effective by Dr. Paul Farmer in earlier studies in

Haiti, where the partners were called *accompagniers*. It seems that Ranko and his wife had devised their own system of reminders using their cell phones.

HAART drug resistance that allows HIV to spread most effectively in the bodies of patients on therapy usually follows specific patterns. AZT and 3TC were two of the three drugs in the first-line therapy in the national Masa program. They were given together as Combivir. In 2008 the program switched from Combivir to Truvada, which is a single pill containing the two drugs emtricitabine and tenofovir, because it seemed to have fewer toxic side effects. In both regimens, the third drug used was usually efavirenz. Efavirenz, however, was not used in women who might be pregnant, as it was thought to be potentially dangerous for the fetus. In women of childbearing age it was usually replaced with nevirapine, which, along with AZT, is also one of the drugs often used to reduce mother-to-child transmission of HIV.

Most of these drugs attack the same part of the virus, the reverse transcriptase enzyme, which is needed for this virus to produce its progeny. They include the nucleoside- or nucleotide-analogue drugs that work by mimicking the DNA molecules that must be inserted when the enzyme makes the DNA copy. Nucleoside-analogue reverse transcriptase inhibitors (NRTIs) include AZT or ZDV (zidovudine), d4T (stavudine), DDI (didanosine), 3TC (lamivudine), TNF (tenofovir), and FTC (emtricitabine). The drug AZT shares complete drug resistance with d4T, and 3TC shares complete drug resistance with FTC. So if a patient becomes resistant to one, the other is also useless. Some other reverse transcriptase inhibitors, such as NVP (nevirapine) and EFV (efavarinz), are not nucleoside analogues and are designated NNRTIs (non-nucleoside reverse transcriptase inhibitors). They, too, share complete drug cross-resistance patterns, so one cannot be used to replace the other. Typical three-drug regimens used to treat patients in Africa would include two NRTIs that work through different drug-resistance patterns, such as AZT and 3TC (often given in one pill, as Combivir), and one NNRTI, such as NVP. Recently, the three-drug combination of TNF and FTC (given in one pill as Truvada) and EFV has also become popular.

Newer classes of drugs that attack other parts of the virus, such as the protease enzyme, have thus far been used only rarely in Africa. (The HIV needs its protease to produce mature virus particles.) The drugs that attack the protease are usually two to three times more expensive than standard antiretrovirals. Other newer drugs are also theoretically available, such as those that prevent HIV from inserting itself into the person's chromosome, or those that act by preventing the step during infection when the virus fuses to the immune cell. But these drugs may cost five to ten times as much as AZT or 3TC. It is highly unlikely that they will be used very much in Africa unless special pricing becomes available.

Tlotlo states that she is now on a Truvada-based drug combination. She may also be receiving a protease inhibitor such as lopinavir/ritonavir (sometimes called Kaletra or Alluvia) because she had drug resistance to efavirenz. Drug combinations such as Alluvia have been developed to be more heat stable, so that they will not lose efficiency when used in hot climates where there is a lack of home refrigeration. This drug is probably used in Tlotlo's case because it is possible that she could get pregnant, and she is resistant to nevirapine. In fact, quite a few women with AIDS who were saved from death by HAART have subsequently become pregnant. If they remain on their medication, it serves the dual purpose of treating them and preventing infection in their newborn children. Nevertheless, counseling about birth control would seem to be important for all women who are HIV infected.

The effectiveness of AIDS therapy is obviously judged by whether the ill patient begins to feel well, returns to usual activities of work or parenting, and continues to feel healthy for prolonged periods. At the medical diagnostic level, this is closely associated with the elevation of CD4 lymphocyte numbers, which should be evaluated periodically for everyone on therapy. An assessment of viral load or quantity may also be done, as this test is the first indicator of whether drug resistance is present, and whether a new drug combination is working effectively. However, the VL test is expensive, so it is not likely to be used very often in Africa.

Sarah had a CD4 count of five when she was finally put on antiretroviral drugs. This is extremely low. It means that about 99 percent of her immune lymphocyte cells had already been destroyed by the HIV in her body. When the immune-cell destruction is so severe, recovery becomes more difficult—although even such severely ill patients usually survive and recover. When ARV treatment programs such as Botswana's begin, triaging may be done, with patients who have the most advanced illness being treated first. At that time, success rates may be a bit low, but as the programs progress to the treatment of patients who are not yet debilitated, overall survival rates increase.

In cities such as San Francisco or Paris, where many AIDS patients have been on HAART for ten to fifteen years, rates of drug resistance seem higher than in Africa. This is particularly important for new infections. If newly infected people get infected with drug-resistant strains of HIV, the standard drugs will not work, whether used for AIDS therapy or for the prevention of mother-to-child transmission. For malaria and TB, drug resistance has become so common that it is now the biggest impediment to progress with those diseases. We must hope that this does not happen with HIV in Africa. Careful monitoring and surveillance of new infections in sites where AIDS therapy has been used the longest, such as Gaborone, will be important for guarding against this possibility.

Ranko had TB before the AIDS epidemic began, in 1979. It was apparently treated successfully. In 1989 he had a malaria-like illness, which he now believes might have been caused by the acute phase of HIV infection. This is logical. In any case, it should not have been malaria, as this disease is rare in southern Botswana. In 1999 he had clinical AIDS, with another bout of TB, which could have occurred after a slow, ten-year destruction of his immune system. Sarah had a diagnosis of cervical cancer, a type of cancer that may also arise and grow more rapidly in women who have had their immune system destroyed by HIV.

Ranko, it would appear, is a survivor. As a child, he somehow avoided an evil uncle who tried to kill him to acquire his inherited cattle. Thus far he has navigated a similarly treacherous course imposed by HIV. He was saved the first time by a sympathetic maternal grandfather. He was saved the second time by the availability of effective drugs to control and reverse progression of his HIV/AIDS.

The Page Is Turning Red

Blood Transfusion as a Risk for HIV Infection

IT ALL STARTED with a simple enough procedure, the insertion of the then-popular IUD called the Copper T. The twenty-nine-year-old new mother had decided on a stop-gap method of birth control while she still pondered tubal ligation. With three children under eight years old and a new legal business to run, a more permanent solution had to be found. She often joked that she was the most fertile woman on earth; that her husband just had to look at her askance and her belly would start to rise.

She was a bit weary of surgery though. Her first child had been delivered by cesarean section when she was only twenty-one, and iodine deficiency during her second pregnancy had led to surgery to excise an overactive goiter: two major surgeries in her relatively young life.

She had no experience with a Copper T, and although the process of insertion was a bit unpleasant, she was off the examining table within minutes and in time for a business meeting. Two weeks later, she was consulting her GP, having spiked her toe with a garden implement, and she made the joke that since she was paying by the hour, she might as well extend the examination by inviting him to check her newly inserted IUD. The doctor obliged, and then with a frown on his face he announced that there was no evidence of an IUD.

Within a couple of days, it was determined that the gynecologist who had inserted the IUD had spiked it right through the wall of the uterus, stapling it firmly onto her intestine.

"What a mess!" the GP whispered under his breath.

"What does this mean?" Amelia asked in alarm. A new baby and a new business were already a taxing mix; she could not deal with extended hospital stays. Where could the IUD have gone? When she had first visited her GP she had expected to leave with a bandaged toe, in time to finish work in her struggling garden that same afternoon. She had since then, though, been X-rayed, examined, and reexamined.

The year was 1988, and there was a new doctor at the main referral hospital who used a nifty little technique called laparoscopy; he would not only retrieve the errant IUD, he would also tie off those egg-producing fallopian tubes. All without opening Amelia up with a major incision!

"I have just had an operation on my neck. I don't want another operation. Can't you pull out the Copper T?"

"I am sorry. The device went clean through the wall of the uterus. The only way to retrieve it is through surgery. But don't worry. This is not the old kind of surgery."

"I have a business to run. I have been away too long as it is. My business is going to collapse."

"You will be out of this hospital in two days. I promise."

Doctors and nurses had always marveled at what they called Amelia's high threshold for pain. When she was in labor with her latest child, it was she who had asked for more time to try for natural birth, when the attending doctor and the nurses suggested that perhaps she should be prepared for a cesarean section. She thought that perhaps that explained why the gynecologist had been able to thrust a sharp object right through the wall of her uterus with only a little whimper from her, and why she had not felt much discomfort even afterward. She might have a high threshold for pain, but she was scared of blood and cuts and wounds; she was not keen on being cut up for the third time.

With the assurance that the laparoscopy procedure meant a small incision, through which not only would the IUD be retrieved but also her tubes could be tied, Amelia submitted herself to the doctors once again. The nurses marveled at her decision to have a tubal ligation at her age; it was an operation that was often recommended by foreign medical doctors, only to be rejected by women, no matter how many children they may already have had.

On the third day after the operation, the doctor with the amazing new technique was rather miffed to see Amelia still in the hospital.

"What is she doing here? There is no reason for her to still be here."

"She says she is in pain."

"She should not be in pain"

"I am in pain. And there was a small bead of pus on the site of the incision. Is that a problem?" Amelia had asked the nurse to raise the issue of the pus with the doctor but she had not. His brisk pace and butterfly kind of landings at the various beds did not allow for extended discussions about each patient. And the nurse's English, although very good, was still her second language, used only from 7:30 AM to 5:00 PM. She was reluctant to start conversations that would call for extensive use of English.

"I was speaking to the nurse, Miss." The doctor was firm in his rebuke. He was not used to talking directly to the patients. The doctor felt somehow disrespected.

"But I don't feel well."

"We do not have room for you to spend the whole year here!"

"Why would I want to stay in this place?"

"You are fine! The operation was a success."

"It went well? I understand the IUD broke. That only a piece was removed."

"Yes, but that is not a problem. Tissue will build around the piece left inside, and with time, it will be part of your body." The doctor had darted the nurse an ugly look. It was clear that he had not expected Amelia to know about the broken IUD.

Amelia was too weak to argue or ask more questions. Or perhaps she was simply too scared to find out more. A piece of copper becoming part of her body was not her idea of a successful surgery. Her mind kept on going back to the new baby she had to take care of and the new business she had to run. She had staff to pay, and every day in the hospital would have significant financial implications.

The nurses, too, seemed to have some concerns, but the doctor had spoken and sure enough, Amelia was discharged from the hospital that same day, with an array of medications to take at home.

"What is this?" Amelia was examining one particular bottle of pills with suspicion.

"This is to help you sleep." The doctor explained impatiently.

"I can't take Valium. It gives me nightmares."

"This is diazepam. Not Valium." The young lawyer was taxing the doctor's patience. She was asking too many questions. Amelia had overheard the doctor muttering something about patients who thought they knew everything. Amelia did not think she deserved this label; if anything, she had been very careful not to come across as arrogant or obnoxious. Notwithstanding the confidence of the doctor that she was fine, Amelia felt that something had gone horribly wrong with the surgery.

That night, Amelia had one of her most fantastic nightmares; she was hurtling through space, dodging moons, suns, and celestial beings, unable to land safely because she was piloting a spaceship constructed out of lace. She was afraid it would disintegrate on impact. She screamed as she landed it back on earth. She had always had spectacular dreams, but this diazepam-induced one, as a Copper T nestled out of reach in her belly, was in a class of its own. She learned, of course, that Valium and diazepam were one and the same thing. The doctor had not believed her when she said she could not take the drug.

More importantly though, within a week Amelia was back in the hospital. A ball of pus the size of a peach had ballooned at the site of the laparoscopy incision. Within hours of readmission she was babbling away, under the influence of drugs, telling a ward full of patients and anyone who cared to listen her life story, including quite a few intimate details. Many who listened clucked with sympathy; she was not expected to live. A few days later, when she was moved to a smaller ward, a cleaning woman, finding her bed empty, assumed that she had died, and felt obliged to spread the terrible news of the death of the young woman who had left behind three children and a sad-looking husband.

In her new ward, pus oozed from her side and she stank like a dead donkey. Her wardmate had to be moved to another room; she could not take the stink and Amelia's writhing from the pain. Visitors tried, out of politeness, not to wrinkle their nose from the stench. Pity welled in their eyes. Her husband kept her informed about the kids at home, and when he thought they could take it, he got them to peek through the window to talk to their mother. The baby had had to go off the breast.

After more than a week of being hooked to a catheter and all manner of contraptions, Amelia decided to try standing up and walking across the room while the nurses where not looking. She needed to test her strength. She walked gingerly to the end of the room, but as she walked back to the bed her bandage was torn off from the pressure of the pus behind it, and yellow, red, and purplish goo erupted from the gaping wound, spattering on the floor. She looked down at her prunelike feet, stained by her own rot, and wondered about the protocol of dealing with one's own decay. Was she expected to clean it up? It seemed rude to just climb back onto the bed, leaving that nasty mess on the floor. And there was a nurse who was always complaining of overwork and underpay; she was not going to be happy. Amelia was shuffling to the bathroom to get cleaning materials, with a hand clamped against the wound, when one of the more sympathetic nurses came in, assisted her back to the bed, and took off her cute little lacy satin nightdress. Amelia noted that the nightdress was soaked in blood and puss. It was as if an angry painter had tried to obliterate the beauty of the blue, purple, and pink flowers on the garment with similar colors. And the smell!

"What was she doing off the bed?" Dr. Laparoscopy demanded when he was called to attend to the emergency.

"She has been on the bed for more than a week. I think it's good that—"

"She needs blood. Order some blood for transfusion."

"No!" Amelia's voice was clear.

"No?"

"No blood. I would rather take months to recover than have a blood transfusion."

The doctor and the nurse exchanged looks as he left the room. It was only later that Amelia learned that not only had Dr. Laparoscopy broken off the T part of the Copper T, leaving the rest of the device in her intestine, but he had also left a swab buried in her body; thus the infection that nearly claimed her life. What was clear, though, was that his earlier arrogance had been a little tempered. Indeed, when after four weeks in the hospital, Amelia demanded a day off to be with her family, the doctor indicated that while he could not officially sign her out, he would not stop her if she tried to go. So thin that the only item of clothing that would fit her was a long skirt pulled up to serve as a shoulder-baring dress, and supported by her sister and husband, Amelia ventured out of the hospital for a day's visit with family.

It was perhaps the secret of the forgotten swab that made it possible for Amelia to prevail on the issue of the blood transfusion. Or perhaps it was simply that in mid-1988, the question of whether to transfuse or not was not always an easy one to answer. Blood could kill just as it could save.

Amelia recalls 1988 as the year the pages started to turn red. She had never herself been a blood donor, on account of her abhorrence of bleeding, but she had always accompanied her husband when he gave blood, often only as far as the car park and occasionally as far as the front office. The visits, though, had gotten her interested in HIV/AIDS, and by the time of her surgery she knew about the three-month "window period" during which HIV might be missed, and the panic setting in at the Red Cross Blood Bank. She had joined one of the Red Cross HIV/AIDS counselors in mounting education campaigns.

"The page is turning completely red!" the Red Cross counselor had pronounced with alarm.

Over the months since the Red Cross had incorporated HIV/AIDS pre- and posttesting in the blood collection process, steadily but surely the red + used to indicate HIV-positive status had assumed a more prominent place on the records. The facility's main function was the provision of safe blood to hospitals, and the increasing incidence of positive HIV testing meant that the Red Cross was discarding blood at an unprecedented rate.

A successful blood bank profiles its potential donors carefully, ensuring that the targeted population is generally healthy and that blood collection is done as efficiently as possible. One population of choice had always been soldiers, strong, healthy young men who could be found in one location. But by the end of 1987, the previously occasional red + had started to show up too often for the blood bank to ignore. Something had to be done. It was not enough to simply discard the tainted blood; the donors had to be engaged somehow. What is more, discarding blood without informing the donors meant that the donors would keep coming back to donate blood without knowing that it was a waste of time and resources, as their blood was destined for destruction. The mandate of the facility had to be extended to include HIV testing as well as pretest and posttest counseling, and it might even be argued that blood collection started to be undermined by the demands of HIV testing.

The blood bank had to look for a new pool of donors, and it looked to high school students. They were younger and could be expected to have shorter track records of sexual activity. With time though, even with this group the pages started to steadily turn red.

"We have to go to primary schools!"

"But they are smaller, literally! We can not extract the pint of blood we need!"

"Well, we will have to extract less then!"

"What about the ethics? Do we have to get consent from the parents?"

"What about the ethics of failing to save lives?"

"We can't!"

"We have to!"

"We need to expand our HIV/AIDS testing capacity!"

"There is still the window period to worry about."

"We need to profile our individual donors better."

"We need to educate the public."

One of the counselors recalls a faithful blood donor who refused to stop donating even after being informed of his HIV-positive status. What is more, he promptly made arrangements to marry his long-time girlfriend, the mother of his three sons. He expected to die within a couple years and he wished to provide financial security for his family. The message and the reality then were that AIDS killed. The counselor attended the man's wedding with a mixture of emotions. She understood the donor's declared motives, but she could not help but feel that the donor was also motivated by the need to ensure that he would have a nurse to take care of him, when the time came. After all, men are told all the time, "Get married! If you do not, who will take care of you when you are old or ill?" The counselor watched as the beaming wife took her vows, totally oblivious to the implications of the swollen lymph nodes giving her partner of fifteen years a rounded face.

"Could her death be read from those nodes?" the counselor wondered to herself. Too many questions still remained unanswered.

"Do I have an obligation to inform the wife about her husband's HIV-positive status?"

"Do I have the authority to refuse to pass him on to the blood extraction team?"

"Do I have the obligation to inform the rest of the team?"

During those years when the pages turned red, the questions were numerous and ethics clashed, demanding careful balancing.

Amelia is still carrying the long part of the Copper T within her, but she is free of HIV—thanks, in large measure, to that early encounter with the counselors at the Red Cross Blood Bank.

✦

Difficult medical procedures sometimes lead to difficult decisions concerning blood transfusion. Red blood cells supply oxygen. White blood cells, including the T lymphocytes that get attacked by HIV, provide a major defensive barrier against invading germs of all types. Some of these white blood cells attack invading bacteria, especially those that cause purulent infections, such as the abdominal abscess that rapidly developed in Amelia. When her IUD penetrated her intestine, it broke the barrier that normally protects the reproductive organs, as well as the liver, kidneys, and other organs, from the bacteria in the gut. While the internal organs are ordinarily clean and sterile, the gut is a teeming brew of numerous types of pathogens waiting for an opportunity to invade. The copper wire served as a wick, an invitation for the bacteria to invade a site where they're normally unable to go.

A major purulent infection of this type can rapidly spread to the blood, which in turn distributes the bacteria all over the body. Fever occurs, and supplies of blood-cell reinforcements to replace those that attack the invading bacteria are rapidly depleted. Only the bone marrow can produce more cells—both leukocytes to fight the infection and red cells to provide oxygen. When the bone marrow can't keep up, the physician resorts to replacement blood in the form of a transfusion. Many medical events may require transfusions, ranging from trauma and childbirth to malaria.

Before the AIDS epidemic, it was known that transfused blood could carry dangerous viruses, such as hepatitis B. Soon after clinical AIDS was first diagnosed in the United States, it was clear that the cause could be transmitted by blood. This was even before HIV was identified. Epidemiological studies revealed that blood-transfusion recipients, injection drug users, and hemophiliacs all had an elevated risk of developing AIDS. Injection drug users essentially got many "minitransfusions" when intravenous needles and syringes containing heroin were passed around, along with residual blood from the previous users. Hemophiliacs had very high rates of HIV infection before methods were available to screen blood, as each hemophiliac received protein-clotting factors derived from hundreds of blood donors. Their chances of receiving HIV-contaminated components were very high.

When whole blood or blood cells are transfused from an HIV-infected individual, the process of transmission is extremely efficient. Virtually everyone who receives a pint of infected blood becomes infected. Those who receive concentrated blood cells from an HIV-infected donor are also almost certain to be infected. Cell-free plasma, sometimes used as a source of antibodies, is less dangerous, especially if it is processed properly.

Tests for detecting HIV in blood were available within a year or two after HIV was discovered, by about 1985. The standard tests most commonly used are relatively inexpensive and very valuable, but by no means perfect. They are based on the detection of antibodies to the virus, not the virus itself. The test kits use various visual markers, such as the + "turning red on the page," to indicate that HIV antibodies are present in the blood being tested. However, it usually takes one to three months for a newly infected person to make the antibodies. If the person's blood is tested during this time, it scores as negative although it is infected and dangerous—a false negative result. Additional tests can be used to cover most—but not all—of this window of "false negativity." The first available procedure for this early window period was an antigen test, designed to detect the protein pieces of the virus. But this test was often ineffective. The best test currently available is based on the direct detection of viral genes by means of a polymerase chain reaction, the highly sensitive test that detects specific gene sequences. However, the PCR tests to detect false negatives were not generally available until the middle 1990s, and they are much more expensive. For this reason, they are still not used in most situations in Africa. Donated blood can be pooled and then tested by PCR to reduce costs, but this is often impractical for logistical reasons, especially in small hospitals.

Blood-test results can also be categorized as false positives, but this is very rare. Those who participated in experimental HIV vaccine trials, for example, may develop antibodies from the vaccine even though they are not infected. Volunteers who participate in such trials are therefore given a card to carry with them that indicates an HIV-antibody test of their blood should not be considered as a true positive unless it is backed up by a PCR test. As we have seen, babies born to HIV-positive mothers also would usually test as false-positive because of the antibodies acquired from the mother. (Some of the babies may actually be infected, but obviously a baby's blood would never be used for transfusion anyway.)

The recognition that blood testing was not perfect led some physicians and some informed patients, such as Amelia, to resist the use of transfused blood whenever possible. Anemic patients would often be allowed to take longer to recover through the slow generation of cells by their own bone-marrow production apparatus. Patients planning to undergo elective surgery would sometimes bank their own blood ahead of time, to be used if needed. Designated donors—friends or family members of the patient—were sometimes recruited. However, they needed to match the patient's blood type, so this was often impractical. Additionally, designated donors often seemed to be just as likely as the general public to be infected with HIV.

The profiling of donors was also an issue. In the early 1980s, donors in the United States and Europe were often paid, and those who donated for payment were more likely to be infected. For efficiency, groups of police officers, military personnel, and employees at large institutions were often the target of blood drives in Africa and elsewhere, but such individuals were also more likely to be infected. Men who work in positions of power and influence may have more sexual partners, and thus a greater risk of being infected with HIV. Younger schoolchildren would obviously be less likely to have had as many sexual experiences, and thus offer a safer source of blood.

The HIV testing of blood donors in the late 1980s, at the time of Amelia's illness, posed numerous ethical problems. Would the donors be notified, counseled, subjected to the risk of being stigmatized? This was way before the network of Tebelopele centers for HIV testing and counseling was established. In 1988, long before drugs were available to treat AIDS in Africa, knowing they were HIV positive would have been of no benefit to donors, only to their partners or family members. AZT, the first AIDS drug, was just beginning to be used in 1988. At best, it extended life by just a year or so. Only when triple-drug HAART combinations became available five to six years later could HIV patients be helped very much, and treatment for most Africans with AIDS is still not available. Units of HIV-positive blood were sometimes donated for research, but this also posed ethical problems unless the donors were asked about this possibility before they donated. Many feared that the establishment of a procedure to inform donors about their HIV status would scare potential volunteers from donating. Even though learning of one's positive status had no direct benefit to HIV-positive individuals, in the late 1980s and early 1990s the blood banks were often the only places where people could learn their HIV status. This made some worry that volunteers who suspected they were infected would give blood to find out. If they did, it would create another category of high-risk donors.

Until now, Botswana has had no medical school. A minority of the resident physicians are citizens who trained elsewhere and came back. The majority are foreigners on two- to three-year contracts. This poses additional challenges in communication, as few speak Setswana. Presumably the physician who treated Amelia, who was both arrogant and incompetent, would not be practicing today. Medical malpractice has long been a legal specialty in the United States, and obstetricians and gynecologists are among the most vulnerable doctors. But such controls on physicians were nonexistent in Botswana in 1988 and remain nonexistent in most of Africa today.

Fortunately, the transmission of HIV infection via transfusion of blood or blood products is now quite unusual, especially in countries that have provided adequate resources to address the problem. Improvements are still needed in many African countries. Perfection—to eliminate all risk—will never be possible so long as blood transfusions still occur.

A Tribal Tradition

Male Circumcision to Prevent HIV Infection

MAISAKOMA, MASOSWE, MADINGWANA, Mabusapelo, Mant-shakgosi, Malomakgomo, Majekere, Mangana, Manoga, and, lastly, Matukwi; the procedure was reinitiated in the 1970s and the last was in 1988. The Bakgatla tribe's chief had relaunched *bogwera* and *bojale,* the age-old initiation ceremonies during which young men were circumcised and both sexes were schooled in matters related to marriage, raising families, and being responsible adults. The ceremonies had not been performed for two decades, as they had been casualties of admission into the tribe of the Christian faith.

Although traditionally an annual event, after relaunching the initiation ceremony, the Bakgatla tribe's chief had never managed to assemble the necessary numbers to justify the creation of a *mophato* (a regiment that goes through the process together), and after years of starts and stops, he finally gave up. There was generally little support from the more educated members of the tribe, who tended to reject traditional practices as backward. The chief was a headstrong man, and it did not help that he could be rather controversial and, on occasion, autocratic. His views had sometimes brought him into conflict with the government. Among the traditional practices he defended were the traditional use of marijuana (especially for medicinal purposes), the practice of *bogadi/lobola,* and the use of corporal punishment for civil infractions of all types. He held strong patriarchal beliefs about the place of men, women, and children in society. But even this deeply traditional man, once all his four children had undergone their respective initiation ceremonies, stopped the practice. The 1988 initiates, therefore, were the last.

Tshepo belongs to the Matukwi Regiment, having gone through the initiation ceremony in 1988. He is the youngest child of seven in his family, the least educated, and the only one of the sons who has undergone the ceremony. He was nineteen at the time. His mother was the one who urged him to do it. She herself had undergone the female ceremony when she was already a grown woman, when the chief had first restarted it. Tshepo's mother also persuaded her daughter, a graduate of a Western university, to go through the ceremony. This was the talk of the village for a while; it was said that Tshepo's mother had raised her daughter well, "See how she obeyed her, when she asked her to go for *mophato.*"

Tshepo, though, was always conflicted about being a member of *mophato.* When he was with members of his *mophato* he felt pride and camaraderie. He had been taught that uncircumcised males remained boys forever and that their sexual prowess would be forever limited by that fact. Circumcised men, on the other hand, were real men who had been taught secrets that could not be shared with boys. In addition, members of a *mophato* were friends and confidants for life. Still, there was always the hint that circumcised men were rural, backward, and uneducated. Tshepo's older brothers, however, never indicated that they considered Tshepo's having gone through the *bogwera* ceremony as in any way setting him apart. That is, not until 2008.

In 2007 the chief died, and a year later his son was installed, with much pomp and ceremony. The regiments were called into action for months as they rehearsed for the installation. Tshepo's pride in his culture knew no bounds. His brothers, the educated ones, were excluded from taking part in the rehearsals. They would join the multitudes of spectators on the actual day, but there was no way they could be allowed to join any regiment, not even just for fun.

On the day of the installation of the new chief, Tshepo woke up to a beautiful September day, with the previous night's war songs still ringing in his ears—until he realized that around him men were getting up with songs already on their lips. They had spent the night camping out with the new chief, and their excitement was palpable. They would usher him into the *kgotla* in a couple of hours, and Tshepo could not wait. He was a man, and he felt strong and confident. He might not have much formal education, but he had the special education qualifying him to play an integral part in the installation of a chief. Many, including members of other tribes, even Western ones, would watch as he sang and danced. He was special. His culture was special.

Two hours later, freshly showered and specially attired in leather sandals, buckskin, and feathers on his head, Tshepo, together with more than two hundred other men, sang his way into the *kgotla* to usher in the new chief. Tshepo watched and listened, singing with the men to punctuate the morning. The speeches by all the others he could have done without; he was waiting for the moment when his new chief would be draped with the leopard skin. He knew that the chief had shot the leopard himself, and that fact filled him with pride. In some tribes, the chief obtained a skin from the Department of Wildlife. Not in his tribe!

Finally the moment came; the chief, regal and stern-faced, was draped with the leopard skin, and the transformation almost brought tears to Tshepo's eyes. The crowd thundered in applause. Praise poems rang in the air. Ululations trilled. The chief's uncle presented him with the other items symbolizing his rule: a club, a spear, and a shield. And then it was the chief's turn to speak.

He urged his tribe to be united and to be proud of what makes it unique and different. And then he made a promise that made Tshepo's heart sing with pride; to restart the tradition of *bojale* and *bogwera,* a central part of which is male circumcision. The ululations rang out. As the noise died down, Tshepo thought he heard the chief link the age-old Bakgatla tradition of regimenting the society into agemates for education, cooperation, and mutual assistance, to the circumcising of males to prevent HIV infection. He was confused. When was an African traditional practice ever linked with anything good? Wasn't HIV infection linked to "harmful traditional practices"?

A month later, the chief came to his small village to address a *kgotla* meeting, and he repeated what Tshepo thought he had heard. *Bogwera* was going to be reintroduced and this time with the assistance of doctors and scientists—all this as part of Botswana's fight against the spread of HIV. He still did not understand, but he was proud that he was part of a select few. He had tested negative for HIV a year before and he wondered whether he had *bogwera* to thank for that.

❈

Historically, male circumcision was done in many tribes in Africa before missionaries introduced Christianity and discouraged pagan rituals. But instead of conducting the surgery on newborn infants, as now occurs in Western cultures, it was part of the initiation into adulthood.

For at least a decade, a few anthropologists have reported that lower rates of HIV infection seem to occur in geographical regions where male circumcision is practiced. But this association was by no means perfect and was often confused and confounded by the link between circumcision and other religious or cultural practices that were also associated with sexual behavior. To test the hypothesis, several controlled trials were conducted in Uganda, Kenya, and South Africa. Young adult males were circumcised, and the rates of new HIV infections among them were compared with those of uncircumcised males living under the same conditions. The results were conclusive. Male circumcision offered a 50 to 60 percent protection rate against HIV infection when an uninfected man had vaginal sex with an HIV-infected woman.

Current rates of circumcision are quite low—perhaps 10 percent—in southern Africa, where the HIV epidemic is severe. In Muslim countries in West Africa, where male circumcision rates are high, rates of HIV infection are much lower. In Western countries, where males are circumcised at high rates as infants, the practice is associated with better hygiene and lower rates of some sexually transmitted diseases, such as genital ulcers.

When men are circumcised as teenagers or adults, it is extremely important that they refrain from sex until the surgical wounds have completely healed. Failure to do so can increase the risk of HIV infection when the integrity of the penile skin is impaired. If circumcised men are already HIV infected at the time of the procedure—whether or not they know they are infected—and they engage in sex before their circumcision wounds have healed, this will increase the risk that the female partner also gets infected. It is particularly important to realize this, because policy guidelines sometimes recommend that HIV-infected men should be offered the procedure, to avoid stigma and discrimination. If HIV-infected men were denied the surgery and it became standard practice for uninfected men, it obviously could become an inadvertent marker of infection.

Why should male circumcision provide such protection? A logical reason is that the penile foreskin, which is removed and discarded, is the richest source of cells that are susceptible to infection during sexual exposure. A specialized type of immune cells, called Langerhans cells, provide a target for infection both on the penis and in the female vagina. In the Merck vaccine trial, in which some volunteer participants appeared to have a greater risk for infection, it might be important to note that those with the increased risk were uncircumcised males.

Tshepo's mother, who encouraged him to undergo the *mophato* ceremony, had undergone a tribal initiation ceremony herself, and she persuaded her daughter to do the same. But the female initiation did not include genital mutilation, sometimes also called female circumcision. This procedure, practiced in some African countries, is dangerous and certainly would do nothing to protect the woman against HIV.

When researchers in Botswana asked adult men if they would undergo circumcision if it would offer them partial protection against HIV, most men surveyed indicated that they would. Since the news about the benefits of the procedure, there have been long waiting lists of men who are anxious to have it done. A challenge for health authorities is to mobilize an adequate number of health practitioners to provide the surgery. The procedure should be performed by experienced experts using sterile techniques, as adverse complications can occur. The circumcision of male infants is of course more ideal, and it is also being promoted much more vigorously in Africa. Yet the benefits from this practice for reduction of HIV infection will take twenty to thirty years to appreciate, when the infants have grown into adult men and have been sexually exposed to HIV.

At the tribal ceremony in 2008, the enlightened new chief announced his intent to reestablish the *bogwera* tradition. But this time experienced surgical experts would be involved. And because the new chief reigns in a time when the AIDS epidemic is rampant in the area—which wasn't the case before 1984—the benefits will be much greater. An astute leader is combining the results of modern medical research with an ancient cultural practice, for all the right reasons.

A Matter of Commitment

Development of an HIV Vaccine

CUPS ARE CLINKING AROUND US as a group of tourists are served their coffee. They are animated; they have just returned from the Okavango Delta, arguably one of the most breathtaking places in Africa, perhaps the world. It has been a particularly dry year, so I can just imagine the congregation of game in and around the Chobe River, before the rains come and pools are created all over the game park, causing the animals to disperse. I am eavesdropping, half listening to the stories of elephants, leopards, and lions, when Lebang arrives, and he almost walks past before his questioning eyes are met by acknowledgment from mine.

"Mr. Lebang?"

"Yes. I thought it was you."

"Have we ever met?" This a question I ask all the time, for in my line of work you meet many people. You are bound to forget faces and names, resulting in embarrassment.

"No, we have not. But of course I know who you are."

Lebang accepts an offer for a soft drink but declines offers of anything else. The tourists get up and move to the pool area of the Gaborone Sun Hotel, and Lebang and I continue with our interview. I am determined to guess the age of this good-looking, neat, compact man. I decide that he must be about thirty-five years old. That would be the average in Botswana, when a man has just recently married. I imagine that if he has children they will be around five years old. Why would a man with preschool kids—a period when parents, especially working parents, can hardly be persuaded to be engaged in any activity not involving children—sign up for a vaccine trial? Maybe he is not married. In which case, one would expect him to be pursuing the rectification of that situation, for no doubt his relatives are on his back.

"Was it hard for you to decide to sign up for the HIV-vaccine trial?"

"For me, once I heard about the vaccine trials and heard that volunteers were being invited to come forward, I just had to go. I have always donated blood and whenever there is a blood shortage, I get called. I just think that that is what every responsible citizen should do."

"What did your family think?"

Lebang explained that the first time he went to the Botswana-Harvard Partnership, where the trial was being conducted, he went with his wife. They had discussed the call for volunteers and had decided they would both enroll as candidates. Later, though, they decided only one member of the family would enroll.

"After that, we told our children. Our twin boys are twenty-one years old and our younger son is sixteen years old. They understood that it was something that had to be done because we explained why it was important."

Lebang says that his parents, too, understood that it was only through the sacrifices of volunteers like their son that a vaccine for HIV might be found, although at first they were fearful.

"But you are HIV negative. Why would you care?"

I was challenging him.

"It is precisely because I was negative that I enrolled. I have been donating blood since the eighties, and when HIV became a reality in Botswana, it was logical for me that I should test and encourage others to test. I am always encouraging people to test. I talk to my friends and relatives and I encourage them to test. Afterward, even those who are positive thank me for that. It is better to know your health status than not to know."

Lebang says that he goes for regular medical checkups and never waits to be ill before making routine yearly appointments. He goes on to explain.

"I am very aware of my body. I know when something is wrong because I eat right and exercise regularly. For example, I was able to tell the doctors, who did not believe me at first, that there was something wrong with my gallbladder. I know my body and I know when something is wrong."

With the information that he had twenty-one-year-old twins, I knew that my estimate of his age was way off. It turned out that he was forty-six years old. His favorite exercise, he said, was walking, and he often walked from Gaborone to Shoshong, a distance of more than 200 kilometers.

"Why?"

"I love nature and the solitude."

"Did you ever regret enrolling in the program?"

"No, no. Never! I believe in commitment. I knew why I wanted to do it, and once I had decided, I was committed to the program. You see, there were people on placebos and others on the real thing. I never felt any difference after the injection, nothing. No dizziness, nothing. And the periodic tests did not show any deterioration in my health. I believe it is because I am a healthy person, generally. I eat well and exercise. That is why I felt confident to take part in the trials. And once I enrolled I followed all their instructions. You have to, otherwise the good intentions of the scientists will come to nothing. There were people who enrolled and then left. That is not good."

I wanted to know whether his wife shared his views, and he was confident that she did.

"That is why we went together, and that is why I could sign up for a process that was to take twelve months. Later I learned that I was not on placebo but on the real thing, but I was not worried. I am very happy I took part because this AIDS problem needs all of us to take part. That is just the way it is."

"How do you explain your HIV-negative status in a country that has such a high prevalence rate?"

"I believe in taking care of myself, in good health. And, because I tested early on and tested negative, that gave me the incentive to stay negative. When you are negative, you want to stay negative. That is why I encourage people to test."

About twenty-five years ago, the secretary of health and human services for U.S. president Ronald Reagan announced that the cause of AIDS had been found. The epidemic was expanding at frightening speed. Without the knowledge of what caused AIDS, scientists had not known how the epidemic could be controlled. Now that the apparent cause had been identified, she said, a protective vaccine should be available in a few more years. Some public health policy officials and medical scientists assumed that a safe and effective vaccine could easily be made and would become available soon. Such vaccines had been made for a wide range of other viral diseases, such as measles, mumps, rubella, polio, and influenza. One of the first vaccines ever made, for smallpox, had even succeeded in eradicating the disease throughout the world. With some others, such as the polio vaccine, the disease was almost eliminated. For most viral diseases, good vaccines had been made, but antiviral drugs were thought to be much more of a challenge. The opposite turned out to be true in the case of HIV.

Viruses, as obligative intracellular parasites, use much of the production machinery of human cells to produce progeny. They copy their own genetic information but need living cells to supply everything else. Some viruses will grow in cells from different species, such as rabies transmitted by dogs or encephalitis viruses transmitted by mosquitoes. HIV, however, will reproduce itself only in human cells. Bacteria, in contrast, are large enough to carry their own production machinery and thus avoid dependence on human cells for most of the steps needed for reproduction. So antibiotic-type drugs for bacteria in diseases ranging from syphilis to pneumonia were much easier to make than antiviral drugs.

For the pharmaceutical industry, the development of drugs may represent a better "market opportunity" than vaccines, for generating shareholder profits. This is especially true for drugs that large numbers of patients in rich countries would use daily for many years, such as drugs for high blood pressure, asthma, or mental anxiety. Products for medical conditions that can be controlled but not cured are the most profitable. By 1986 or 1987, it was clear that HIV/AIDS had already spread to about a million people in the United States and Europe. AIDS drugs now represented a potential market opportunity. And for research of this type, including product development, large pharmaceutical companies clearly had much expertise.

All of the effective viral vaccines are based on the principle of injecting a killed or weakened strain of the virus, or a surface protein, to mimic the first step of a natural exposure and elicit antibodies. The viral surface proteins are recognized as foreign, and the body recognizes foreign substances by making antibodies against them. As biotechnology matured in the 1980s, some of the viral surface proteins could be made by genetic engineering. An excellent vaccine of this type was made for hepatitis B.

The availability of the hepatitis B vaccine served to raise another dilemma. The greatest burden of hepatitis B disease is felt in Africa and various countries of Asia, such as China. But the cost of the vaccine was relatively high. In Tanzania and Mozambique, the cost of the vaccine was equivalent to a person's entire annual income. For many years, none of the governments or international agencies could find a way to get the vaccine to those countries where it was most needed. With the rise of HIV infection and AIDS, this dilemma created widespread concern that African populations with the highest rates of HIV might be exploited in the development of a vaccine, by providing subjects for test trials, and then not have access to the vaccine because they could not afford it. Yet to establish that a vaccine will work in the populations where it is most needed—for example, among women in southern Africa infected via vaginal sex—would testing in other populations that were exposed through injection drug use or homosexual activities provide the proper assurance? To complicate matters even more, the viruses causing the HIV epidemics in Africa are different from the HIV-1 subtype B that caused the epidemic in the United States and Europe. So, courageous volunteers like Lebang are needed to establish that any vaccine that might work would also work in the epidemic in his region.

After about twenty years of research, we still have no vaccine for HIV, and most experienced vaccine experts believe it will be another ten to twenty years before we do. The major reason that making a vaccine to prevent AIDS is so difficult is the remarkable ability of HIV to change itself by rapid mutation. During natural infection, the human body does make antibodies against HIV. In fact, the antibodies are made so regularly that they serve as the simplest test for infection with the virus or the diagnosis of AIDS disease. But these antibodies do not protect against disease development, nor do they eliminate HIV from the body, which is what happens when antibodies are made in response to measles, mumps, or rubella. At most, the HIV antibodies made during natural infections may slow down the onset of AIDS. By the time the antibodies are made to a specific protein on the surface of the virus, the virus has changed. So, while the antibodies do attack the HIV that was present a few weeks before, now a new mutant virus dominates. New antibodies are made to the mutant virus, but by then a new mutant has evolved and taken over from the first mutant. This process is called immune evasion. It occurs more rapidly with HIV than with any other virus. This characteristic, along with the ability of HIV to hide its genetic code in the DNA of human immune cells, helps explain why it is so difficult to make a vaccine against AIDS.

The second major reason why it is taking so long to develop an AIDS vaccine is that prolonged trials are needed to demonstrate success. After an experimental vaccine is designed and ready for testing, it is first tried in lab animals, such as mice or guinea pigs, and perhaps monkeys. But at best this will tell the researchers only whether the experimental vaccine can induce any immune response, not a protective response. Only people get infected with HIV, so it is impossible to "challenge" laboratory animals with live HIV to determine if an induced immune response would thwart the infection. Each experimental vaccine design that appears to have potential must be tested on human volunteers.

The first human trials are always done for safety, and they take about two to three years. It was a trial of this type—a phase I trial— that involved Lebang as a volunteer. Typically, roughly two-thirds of the volunteers receive the vaccine injection and about one-third get a sterile placebo fluid. Neither the volunteers nor the physicians and nurses know the code that indicates which people get the actual vaccine. After the trial is completed with numerous lab tests and health exams, a determination is made about whether the vaccine had any toxic effects or caused discomfort. If an experimental vaccine causes anything more than very minor problems, it is dropped from consideration.

If the vaccine passes the phase I trial, it is then tested in a larger population of human volunteers in phase II, to evaluate its ability to induce measurable immune responses, such as antibodies. The phase II trial is also designed to determine which types of immune responses are elicited, and which dose of the vaccine seems optimal to elicit the type of immune response predicted to be effective. The phase II trial may take another three to four years. Again, some of the people get a sterile placebo, and all the participants are closely monitored with health exams and clinical laboratory tests. If those who received the actual vaccine have good immune responses as judged by some preset criteria, and no toxic side effects are observed, the vaccine design can move on to a third trial, to test the vaccine's efficacy: phase III.

While the first safety trial may have enrolled twenty-five to fifty volunteers and the second immune evaluation trial a few hundred, the phase III efficacy trial requires several thousand volunteers. Phase III, which can take another three to five years, provides the first indication of whether or not the vaccine protects. The test is based on simple math and statistics: is the number of infections among people who got the vaccine and then got infected by natural exposure lower than the number of naturally acquired infections in the volunteers who got the sterile placebo? Again, neither the trial volunteers nor those conducting the trial know who got the true vaccine or the placebo. All participants are advised to avoid risky sex and exposure to HIV, but inevitably some exposures—and infections—occur. If the volunteers enrolled in the trial are in a very high-risk population, such as young women in southern Africa, their risk of infection is higher, and so fewer people may be needed for the trial. Another way to evaluate efficacy would be to determine if the vaccine prevented AIDS disease even when it did not prevent HIV infection. This could happen, for example, if the vaccine allowed a low level of HIV expansion in the body but kept the level from getting high enough to result in AIDS disease. This would make the trial even longer, however—much longer. In addition to the three to five years needed to measure infection rates, it would require another six to eight years to allow for the usual lag before HIV causes AIDS.

The first experimental vaccine that completed all the trials was similar in design to the bioengineered vaccine for hepatitis B that worked so well. It was based on a protein on the outer-envelope surface of HIV, designated gp120. It failed. The vaccine was harmless and nontoxic, but ineffective.

The scientists then responded by completely changing their design. Rather than making a vaccine designed to elicit antibodies, they designed the next version to elicit immune attack cells that would kill HIV and HIV-infected cells directly, without antibodies. This represented an entirely new concept at the time, as all available vaccines were based on antibodies. Various designs for this new type of vaccine—designated cytolytic T cell vaccines—were made and tested. One involved the injection of pieces of HIV DNA. Another involved the use of other harmless or inactivated viruses to deliver the pieces of HIV that would be needed to stimulate a protective immune response. One of each of these designs was tested for safety in Botswana—where Lebang was a participant—and both passed the phase I test, proving to be harmless. Unfortunately, neither proceeded to the next phase because they were judged to be unlikely to stimulate an adequate level of immunity.

The first vaccine design of this class to reach the efficacy-trial stage was one made by Merck, using a seemingly harmless human virus that causes the common cold. When used as a delivery system for the HIV pieces, it was modified dramatically so that it couldn't even cause colds. The results, however, were more disappointing than for the antibody-type vaccine. This model, designated adeno 5a, not only gave no protection but also seemed to increase the risk of HIV infection in those who received the vaccine. Adeno 5a was not tested in Botswana. In retrospect, we can speculate about why this vaccine design may have increased the risk of infection. But at a minimum it was a huge disappointment, and almost all the experimental vaccines designed on the same principles had to be discarded.

Vaccine researchers haven't given up, nor should they. They are already actively pursuing totally different strategies based on new biological tricks that did not exist ten or twenty years ago, when the first trial vaccines were designed. But few of these new ideas are even ready for testing in laboratory mice or guinea pigs. And after that they will require ten or more years of testing in people.

Lebang is still a hero. But we will need much more time and many more Lebangs before we have an effective vaccine for HIV. Until then, we must rely even more on other methods of protection from infection—behavior changes, condoms, circumcision of men, and the creative uses of drugs to decrease transmission. No one ever said that the control of HIV would be easy.

· 12 ·

Ancestral Control

Evil Spirits and HIV as the Cause of AIDS

"JUDGE, I AM DYING. I AM DYING." The voice was no more than a whisper, and in the background I could hear other voices.

"Where are you?"

"This is Lemme. I am sick, Judge. I am sick."

"Lemme, where are you?"

"In Orapa. In a hospital. I am dying."

"Why Orapa? Why so far away?"

"I came here so my sister could take care of me. I am sick. I am dying . . ."

There was desperation in the weak voice, but before I could ask any more questions the mobile phone connection went dead. Attempts to call back were futile. I did not know Lemme's sister's name; in fact I had not known she had a sister in Orapa. I also knew that "sister" could mean a close cousin, so finding Lemme's sister's name and number was not going to be an easy matter.

A week later my clerk knocked on my office door and announced, "Lemme wants to see you, Judge."

I was a little surprised that Lemme needed an announcement before she came into my office. I was particularly surprised that she

133

was back in the office before her ten-day sick leave was over. The last time we spoke, she sounded like she was not about to spring out of bed in a few days. And in fact, after the phone call, I had checked with her supervisor and found out that she had asked for an extension of her sick leave.

"Tell her to come in," I answered. I looked up, searching the clerk's face for some indication of Lemme's state of health. That she was really ill was common knowledge. Employees had been dying at an alarming rate during the past two years or so, and any indication of serious illness brought on long faces and whispers among the staff.

"She is downstairs, Judge. She can't walk up. She wants you to go down."

That made me leap off my chair. The one flight of stairs up to our level was hardly taxing, and seventy-something-old judges were taking them every day without complaint. If a thirty-five-year-old security officer could not make it up those stairs, it had to mean that she was in bad shape. In addition, I knew it had to take courage for a security officer to call a judge down from her chambers to meet in a downstairs room.

I hurried down the stairs and headed to the key room, a little corner room, and there, slumped over the small desk, I found a frail shadow of the woman who had been my security officer since she had come to work with me in 2002. Her face was gray, and her eyes were sunken.

She looked up with great difficulty and repeated what she had said to me from 400 kilometers away through a weak mobile connection, "I am dying, Judge."

I leaned over and touched her face and found it to be clammy with sweat. "Why aren't you in a hospital?"

"They gave me water and discharged me. I am dying." I understood that she meant that she had been given an intravenous drip to replace lost fluids.

"What's wrong? What do they say is the matter with you?" I asked. By this time, the words HIV and AIDS were pounding in my brain. What else could it be? Only two years before, I had lost a particularly close cousin to AIDS, and the pain of that loss was still with me. I had seen her flesh under her skin melt away until the skin clung tightly to the bones. By the time she had died, her mouth was set in a permanent mirthless grin. I was imagining the same fate for the young woman currently slumped over the keys to the various offices around us. Some keys were hanging on hooks and they clanked as I leaned over to hear her response. Someone opened the door, offered apologies, and grabbed a set of keys. Otherwise, around us, the office mill turned.

Lemme's illness had not been sudden. It had crept up on her over months, attacking and retreating repeatedly, every attack seeming to be more serious. When she'd had one of her attacks, which took the forms of nausea, flulike symptoms, diarrhea, chest pains, and blistering lips, to name but a few of her complaints, she had missed work for a day here, two days there. During one such absence, her supervisor had come to my office to explain the situation as he and others believed it to be: "Judge, Lemme is ill again."

I looked up, as I could sense there was more behind the simple words.

"Someone must advise her to do the obvious thing." The supervisor seemed to be ambivalent about raising the matter.

"The obvious thing?"

"Well, these things should be a matter for her family, not me . . ." He trailed off until I asked.

"What are you talking about?"

"Yes, Judge. She must accept that she cannot work."

Was Lemme's supervisor hoping for my support in sacking his junior colleague over a few days' absence from work? Both of us knew that it was not an easy matter to dismiss a government employee, for whatever reason. And why would we want to do that? If government service was good at anything, it was good at providing support for staff illnesses. We both knew that in most cases employees did not even have to file a sick-leave form to prove that they had been ill. To suggest that her absences were sufficient cause for dismissal was crazy, at the very least.

"What do you mean?"

"Well, Judge, have you noticed how Lemme gets ill every time she comes to work? But once she takes time off she gets well again. The problem is here at work!"

The man looked at me as if waiting for me to confirm his theory. I was at a loss to understand what he was talking about. Was he suggesting that someone here at the office was bewitching her? That had to be it. But if that were the case, there were ways in which Lemme could resist such supernatural shenanigans without involving her supervisor and me.

"What do you mean?" I asked again.

"Her ancestors do not want her to work. She must do only the work she has been chosen by her ancestors to do! The thing is, she is not willing to accept her chosen path."

Now it was out. Lemme had said a couple of times that she wanted to tell me something about herself, but somehow I had never found the time for that tête-à-tête. Younger women at the court were always coming to me about love matters, career issues, or problems with children, and I had thought it was about one of those issues that she had wanted to speak to me. When she had not pressed for time to talk, I had forgotten about the request.

"So she is a traditional doctor?" I asked.

"Of course! Surely you are aware?" He seemed perplexed that I had been working in close contact with one possessing such great powers, dangerous powers, even, without taking notice.

"I wasn't, actually. But why should she leave her job?"

"Her ancestors want her to do her calling! To heal the sick! Not to do this kind of work!"

It amused me a little that he seemed to suggest that "this kind of work" was beneath Lemme, while he himself seemed to be doing it pretty happily.

It came to me that Lemme had indicated to me on more than one occasion that she was concerned about my safety. She had had dreams that suggested that powerful, jealous forces had been marshaled against me. She had "seen" this in dreams. We are a nation that believes in dreams and their relevance to day-to-day life, so I did not think she was any different from anyone else. After all, my other security officer had once sought me out on a Sunday morning, her day off, to warn me about a dream she had about me in which I was hurt. She believed that if she did not warn me, some harm would befall me. It was for these reasons that Lemme's dreams had not sounded peculiar to me.

After my conversation with the supervisor, I had the talk with Lemme, and she told me the story of how she had found out that she was a healer. As was almost always the case, the realization that she had been chosen to be a healer came to her after she had been plagued by illnesses and sufferings that no doctor, Western or traditional, had been able to cure. She was twelve years old when she was finally diagnosed, and by that time she had dropped out of school. How could she have stayed in school, with snakes appearing to her day and night and spirits seizing her body and sending her into trances any time they wished?

Even after a traditional doctor had diagnosed the cause of their daughter's persistent headaches, trances, silences, screams, and nose-bleeds, to name but a few of her afflictions, her parents had hoped to get her released from the grip of her ancestors. They had wanted her to return to school, so they thought the best way to do that was to enroll her in a healing church. They reasoned that praying and singing hymns would be a good way to harness and control the ancestral spirits that possessed their daughter.

The ancestors were not pleased by this attempt to avoid responsibility, Lemme told me. On the day of her baptism, which had involved complete immersion in a river, the ancestors had yanked her from under the palm of the priest and for twelve days had supposedly kept her under water. When they finally allowed her to surface, her parents had known that there was no way that their daughter could avoid her fate. They took her across the border to Zimbabwe, and for three years she was trained in how to control and use her powers. She learned to recognize the various ancestors who possessed her and to let them communicate through her. It was a tough and grueling course. Twice she tried to run away, and on each occasion she was caught and whipped senseless by her trainers.

It was only after the training that she was able to go back and finish high school.

When we had this conversation, she had been a traditional healer and diviner for more than ten years, and she had performed countless healing ceremonies. Only a week before our conversation, a nurse at the local hospital had engaged her to exorcise evil spirits from her house. The two had spent a long and frightening night during which Lemme had slain powerful evil spirits that had presented themselves in all sorts of forms, including the forms of cats, short men, and eyes floating in dark rooms. Her boyfriend, who had driven her to the house, had been so petrified by the exorcism that he had driven off, leaving her to find her own way home.

At that time, she had explained that her constant illnesses were the result of her absorbing the illnesses she expelled from others. She needed a strengthening ceremony, she said. She planned to have one at the end of the year in her home village.

"You should come, Judge. Since you like to write books, you should write about it."

"Can anyone attend?"

"Yes, it is a public event. All the healers from the area and some from Zimbabwe attend. A cow is killed and we dress up, sing, and dance. We dance for days."

"You say it is a strengthening ceremony?"

"Yes. Once you dance, you go into a trance and your ancestors, one by one, take over your body. You start speaking in his or her voice. You even change clothes, while in a trance, to dress in his or her clothes. I have never met these people, but once I am in a trance, I can be them. You get your power back."

"Are you happy doing this? This healing?"

"I have no choice. If I don't do it, I will get ill, and I will die. So it's not a matter of being happy or unhappy. Even here in Lobatse, sometimes I wake up and I must sing and dance. The ancestors just take over my body. I was born to do this."

"It must be a great burden."

"Yes, it is. I must use my powers for good. I must heal people. I cannot refuse."

"Your supervisor says you should stop working and heal and divine full time."

"No, I have asked the ancestors. As long as I attend strengthening ceremonies at least once a year, I can work. The thing is, sometimes I do not have time. My home village is far, and we must arrange with other healers. That is why sometimes I get so sick."

When I told her, sometime later, about a cobra that had glided into view as I was watching television in my living room, she was sure that I was either a potential healer or that powerful evil forces were being sent to hurt me.

"Judge, why don't you believe?"

"I just think I live next to a hill, that the space under my front door is too high, and I must find a way to have it blocked."

"You don't understand that as the only woman judge, there are those who wish to harm you."

"Lemme, I will be okay."

"Anyway, you are strong. You are protected. I think you have healing powers, you just don't know it."

Now she was slumped over in the key room, in a uniform that had nothing to do with her healing and divining, and I was concerned that she was going to blame another taxing exorcism for her illness.

"Have you had an HIV test?" I asked. Lemme turned her face up, startled by the question. Despite the ravages of AIDS, its evident presence all around us, it was not a question that was asked often, certainly not directly.

"No, I have not." She sounded relieved to have been asked.

"Do you want to?"

"I am afraid."

"It is best to know. There are drugs now. You could get better."

"I don't want to die."

"If you test now and it turns out that you are positive, you can get drugs."

"Judge, will you come with me? I am afraid!" She was crying and snorting, and tears were pooling on the desk on which her head lay.

"Yes. I'm sure Dr. Thabo Moremi will see you. I will call him right away."

I was not sure of anything, since I had not even called to make sure that Dr. Moremi was at work. When I did call, though, he said he would see Lemme that same day.

Within minutes I had informed the rest of my staff that I would be away for the day as I had to take Lemme to see a doctor. With the help of a couple of strong hands, we half carried, half propelled her to my car, and I took her to the Princess Marina Hospital.

Over the course of the next weeks, Lemme was tested for HIV. When she was found to be positive and her CD4 cell count and viral load were determined, she was placed on antiretroviral therapy. But even before she was placed on therapy, just knowing what ailed her seemed to set her on the road to recovery.

On the day I expected Lemme to start her therapy I went to see her, and I found her in her little house, swaddled with blankets on a sofa, watching television and dozing. A woman who introduced herself as her mother was sitting next to her. On the small coffee table were bottles of pills, a pitcher of water, and a glass.

"I want to thank you, my child, for helping Lemme. She told me all about what you have done."

"I am happy she has found help. I understand she starts her antiretrovirals today. You are aware that one of them may give her bad dreams?" I was concerned that Lemme might confuse the dreams brought on by one of the drugs with dreams brought on by spirits and such things. I could just imagine her going into a singing and dancing spree and collapsing from the exertion required for such a ceremony.

"Lemme will not take her medicines today. We must travel to the ancestral hills to ask the ancestors for permission for her to take these drugs."

Uh-oh, I thought to myself. Here we go again!

"What if the ancestors do not give permission? And how will you travel?" I had not seen a vehicle outside, and I did not think she was in a position to go anywhere by public transport. She was hardly in a position to travel by private transport.

When my own cousin was just about to slip away from us, she had grabbed my hand and made me promise to take her to a healer and diviner. I had known that it was futile, but how could I refuse those pleading, dying eyes? We had carried her out, as she groaned in pain, and put her in the back of a Toyota truck for the drive to the diviner's home, some thirty minutes away. The diviner had blamed a jealous workmate and a spurned lover for my cousin's illness. He had read all this from bones he had thrown at our feet. My cousin died a week later. That was in 1996, before the antiretroviral drugs were available in Africa.

This time, antiretroviral drugs were on a coffee table within arms' reach. Lemme could take them now and start on the road to recovery.

"The ancestors cannot make a decision that would harm Lemme. She is their chosen child. I believe the doctor you sent her to. So the ancestors will agree. But they must be consulted so they can bless the medicine."

I knew better than to argue. "How will you travel? Isn't it too far to travel with a sick person?"

"A relative will come tomorrow morning. By tomorrow night, she will start to take these pills. I thank you, my child, for your kindness."

Lemme has been on therapy now for three years. She was back at work within two weeks of starting therapy. She now keeps an eagle eye out for anyone who looks remotely ill and will drag them to my office for a confidential talk.

Toward the end of 2005 she came to my office, and in that gentle voice of hers she half whispered, "Judge, you must speak to Moemo. He is sick. He must understand that he doesn't have to die . . ."

Lemme was very sick in Orapa. She had an extended sick leave. Talk around the court was of AIDS, which had been killing staff members at an alarming rate. With a gray face and sunken eyes, and too weak to get up a flight of stairs, Lemme appeared near death. It usually takes months to reach this level of severe debilitation and cachexia. Patients who have one of many chronic debilitating illnesses, including AIDS, look similar at the final stage, having suffered severe weight loss—sometimes called slim disease—and dehydration. But before the epidemic of AIDS, this final stage was usually seen late in life, not in patients in their twenties or thirties.

A colleague who observed Lemme's deterioration described how she seemed to get worse when at work. He said that her ancestors did not want her to work at the court. They and others believed she was endowed with supernatural powers as a traditional healer, and that the ancestral spirits were attacking her own health because she was not pursuing the career path for which she was chosen.

Lemme was also afflicted with headaches and nosebleeds as a child of twelve. That was presumably not AIDS. At that age, she was probably too young to have been infected sexually, especially when we allow for the multiyear incubation period before symptoms develop. And twelve seems too old for a child to develop the signs of AIDS after infection from the mother. Blood-transfusion transmission or infection due to childhood rape can occur, but these situations would be very unusual at that age.

An attempt at expulsion of the evil demons through religion was considered. This appeared to fail, and Lemme was sent to Zimbabwe for a three-year training course to realize her destined role as a traditional healer and diviner.

Even a local nurse believed sufficiently in Lemme's abilities to ask her to exorcise evil spirits from her house. Her ceremonial activities provided incentive for her commitment to the rituals, but not a solution for her own illness. Lemme's health continued to deteriorate. Judge Dow then confronted her with the reality of AIDS and the importance of being tested for HIV.

Throughout the history of medicine, infectious diseases have been attributed to supernatural intervention or witchcraft. For just as long, religion and traditional healers have been sought out to resolve health problems. The extent of a society's commitment to such avenues is often related to the literacy of the population, especially the literacy among older generations in cultures where elders are deeply respected.

As the true cause of AIDS, the human immunodeficiency virus seems even more clever than the evil spirits. It is far too small to see but has 10,000 letters in its genetic code and a unique way to parasitize human immune cells. HIV uses its genetic code to program the production of nine different proteins in the human CD4 cells that it infects. Several of these HIV proteins are used to protect the virus from destruction. Others are used to rapidly produce millions of HIV offspring. When the rate of progeny-virus production greatly exceeds the ability of the body to replace dead immune cells, clinical AIDS appears and progresses.

All viruses are too small to see, and almost all kill the cells they infect, but most do not infect human immune cells. In fact, no other virus is known to infect these particular human CD4 T cells, the key cells that activate the rest of the body's immune response. HIV does this by attaching an outer-surface projection, called a gp120, to the CD4 receptor, which is found only on a subset of immune cells. This lock-and-key type of reaction leads to another form of binding to a group of coreceptors found on the same cells. A conventional vaccine, if one existed—unfortunately there is none—would be designed to produce antibodies that would cover the virus so it could not attach to the CD4 or the coreceptor.

HIV is also different from simpler viruses in other ways. The genetic code is RNA, but it is rapidly transcribed "in reverse" to become DNA. The HIV DNA integrates itself with, or "sneaks into," the chromosomal DNA of the human cells. Thus, it can "hide" and avoid being recognized as foreign. Other viruses cannot do this.

Some, such as those that cause colds or flu, also have RNA for their genes, but they have no special mechanism to convert to DNA and then hide in the human genes. Others, such as those of smallpox and herpes, are DNA viruses to begin with, but they don't integrate into human DNA, and they don't evolve by rapidly changing their genes like HIV does.

The fact that HIV produces progeny by changing its viral form of genetic material, RNA, to DNA allows it to mutate and diversify faster than any other virus. Recombination, or the trading of parental genes, is also more efficient with HIV. The net result is an explosion of mutants and chimeric progeny viruses. Because the principle of "survival of the fittest" is also true for viruses, those progeny viruses that can best evade bodily defenses, transmission blocks, or drug treatment are the most likely to give rise to the next generation of the virus in an infected person, or the next epidemic in a population.

By best estimates, HIV entered the human population only fifty to a hundred years ago. Organisms evolve according to their generation time and number of progeny. A single HIV routinely has billions of progeny within a day. People, the host species, are at the other end of the spectrum with two to three progeny every twenty to thirty years. With such a difference, we can readily see why HIV is such a formidable foe: it can adapt much faster than we can. The agents of most other infectious diseases have been around much, much longer—in most cases, long enough for generations of people to evolve with some degree of their own genetic resistance. Earlier studies have already revealed a very small fraction of people with a genetic change, called delta 32, that protects cells from infection with HIV. A research project is now under way in Botswana to identify more human AIDS-risk genes, those that increase or decrease the risk of infection. While the results cannot be used to provide people with information about how to choose their mates, they might provide valuable hints about how to make better drugs, or vaccines, or microbicides.

Recognizing how cunning and devious HIV is as a disease agent, perhaps we shouldn't be surprised that some people invoke supernatural forces to help explain that which is so hard to understand. The virus causes disease by targeting and destroying the immune system. As a result, the final pathways to death with AIDS are many and varied. The cause may be bacterial TB, fungal encephalitis, or even a form of cancer, such as Kaposi's sarcoma or lymphoma. The only common characteristic of these diseases may be their dependence on an intact immune system to prevent death. HIV provides the immune destruction.

There are many reasons why we are so sure that HIV is the cause of AIDS. One is the almost perfect association between HIV infection and destruction of the body's immune system. Another is that drugs designed very specifically to attack HIV, and only HIV, allow patients' recovery and long-term survival. Denialists who choose to ignore this evidence may sacrifice the lives of millions of people, if they are in positions of influence. Infected people may not bother to take life-saving drugs. Uninfected people may engage in risky sex and avoid using condoms.

Judge Dow led Lemme to get tested and to be put on appropriate drug therapy for her disease, which was already very severe. Even then, Lemme wanted to consult with her ancestors, to get their permission to take the drugs. Apparently even the ancestral spirits saw the light. They allowed Lemme to take the medicine and survive. Now, three years later, she is doing fine. The evil witches fought a good battle for Lemme, but in the end she won.

· 13 ·

He Died in China

Fear and Stigma

HE DIED IN CHINA a couple of months shy of his thirtieth birth-day, two years after his wife of one year had died, three months after his wife's ex-boyfriend died. Perhaps it was hearing about that last death that had propelled him out of the country: an attempt at out-running death? He left behind a three-year-old daughter, the cutest, smartest little girl you ever saw.

There were rumors of a third man . . . had he died too?

He had lived his life with an urgency and impatience that bor-dered on fury. Right from the start, he was always in a hurry. He was born to an eighteen-year-old mother and with such amazing ease that the nurses didn't have time to wash their hands to receive him. He skipped crawling altogether, sliding on his bottom instead. Even as a baby he was fearless. He was started in school at four, to limit his mischievous exploits to afternoons only. He was five when he licked the glue off his spiteful teacher's postage stamps, rendering them useless, and when he was seven he selected the greenest and ugliest pair of pants in the shop—to prove that he had the right to chose his own clothes. He was six when he ran across the village, covering at least ten kilometers, to be one of the eyewitnesses to an apartheid-inspired car bombing. At ten, not wanting to be treated as the youngest in his class, he added a year to his age by simply convincing the school principal that her records were wrong. At twelve he decided that Macmillan was a nice-sounding name; he had the authorities add it to his birth records; it is unclear how he managed it.

He was curious, adventurous, always full of life, and on occasion just outright outrageous. He was a slight fellow, but he once slapped a big taxi man across the face; the driver had attempted to change the fare on him at the end of the journey, and he was not having any of that. Above all, though, he had a twinkle in his eye and a mischievous grin that could melt hearts; how else would one explain a policeman driving him home, after ticketing him and seizing his car for some traffic infraction?

He could be as exasperating as he could be charming.

He died in China. And he was buried among strangers in a hideously green coffin, but then he always liked green.

"Is daddy dead too?" asked Gofa, Disana's three-year-old daughter, as the family watched news of the devastation brought on by the earthquakes in China in the spring of 2008.

"No, no! Of course not!" Gofa's grandmother was horrified at the suggestion. The girl was only three years old but very intelligent. She missed nothing. The channel was changed.

"But people are dying in China," she insisted.

"But your dad is fine. He sent us a text message to say he is fine. You spoke to him on the phone only yesterday, remember?"

"Oh. Okay. So only the Chinese are dying?"

"Yes, only the Chinese are dying." An adult lie intended to allay the fears of a three-year-old. Her father had been in China for a month then, and he had been sending text messages, e-mails, and occasionally calling. It was true that he was not in danger; he was in Shanghai, far from the earthquake.

Disana did die in China, within four weeks of his daughter's prophetic question.

His death in China had been preceded by many key events, including a heady falling-in-love, a pregnancy, marriage, and bitterness that sometimes threatened to spiral out of control.

The healthy-looking girlfriend had been on ARVs but had kept the information from her besotted boyfriend. They had been inseparable during those early months, and the couple's haste in setting a wedding date was soon put down to the pregnancy.

To avoid detection, she had stopped taking her drugs, and of course that led to the deterioration of her health. A month after the wedding there was no denying that she was ill, and when he tested positive he flipped.

"You—why didn't you tell me? How could you?"

He had the presence of mind to insist that she enroll in the Mother-to-Child Prevention Program. At first she resisted, but after changing health clinics to avoid detection by a nurse she knew at the first clinic, she relented. Her HIV-positive status would have been evident to any one who cared to glance at her gaunt-looking face and occasionally blistering lips. Still, she tried to hide from what was there for anyone to see. And, in response, no one named the monster. There were whispers and furtive glances, but no public acknowledgment. But at least she was back on the drugs and some hope was restored.

Disana and his wife's next two years together were characterized by sadness, desperation, physical fights, and threats of divorce.

Weary of the fights and perhaps riddled with guilt, she decided to die. She said as much, and simply stopped taking her drugs. Disana begged, pleaded, and threatened, but she would not budge. When the time came, she closed herself in a room, allowing only her parents in to feed and bathe her. Slowly but surely she melted away, her skin tightening around her skeletal frame, her lips turning a bright red and then splitting as dehydration set in. Finally, her body simply shut down.

Why didn't she tell him? Why is this not a unique story? Why didn't he protect himself?

After her death he was ravaged by guilt, anger, fear, and desperation. Perhaps he had not tried hard enough to get her to get back on the drugs. Why did she rob him of a future? How was he going to live with this poison brewing in his body? What if the tests had been wrong and his daughter had been infected? He had her retested and said a prayer of gratitude when she was confirmed as HIV negative. He silently thanked the nurse who nagged his wife into the Mother-to-Child Prevention Program.

"Is this just a pimple, or is it the beginning of the end?" he would wonder as he examined his boyish face.

Often he was seized by depression, causing him to lash out at those near him. He was a widower and the father of a two-year-old at age twenty-nine. He was HIV positive and on ARVs. Would he tell his next lover? Why wouldn't he? Would he ever be married again?

Was he doomed to have one child?

He went for counseling. He had been started on ARVs before he was visibly ill because his CD4 was alarmingly low.

Then, just as he was beginning to rise from the depression, he learned of the death of a man with whom he shared something intimate, although they had never met: a past lover and most probably the same HIV strain. Would he be next? Why did the man die? Wasn't he on drugs? Disana stopped taking his own drugs.

"I need to leave this country for a while. I need some space. I have found a job in China; I want to learn Mandarin. That is the language of the future."

"China?"

"Yes, China."

He had made inquiries and found out that his English degree could get him a teaching job in China while he learned Mandarin. China was indeed becoming a favorite destination for those seeking inexpensive goods, and he knew a couple that had built their entire house from materials purchased in China. There were those who were skeptical about his job prospects, but everyone agreed that he did need some time on his own. His parents agreed to take care of his daughter, and an uncle agreed to sponsor the trip. He promised those who were close enough to inquire that he had enough drugs for at least four months.

Within eight weeks, though, he was dead from meningitis. The Chinese authorities were insisting on either a cremation or a burial in China. They did not want the body transported to Botswana.

"It is because of this A. I. D. thing. That is the problem," a Chinese official whispered, pronouncing each letter with unfamiliarity.

"Can you tell me, how is this AIDS thing transmitted?" asked an American man who had been sharing an apartment with Disana. He had driven Disana to the hospital when he first showed signs of confusion, following headaches that Disana had sworn to him had rendered him deaf. The fear in the man's blue eyes was pathetically obvious, but Disana's aunt had a family back in Botswana that was horrified by the prospect of having one of their own buried in some faraway cemetery, so she was not in the mood for educating an adult on matters of HIV infection. The week had been hard; she and her brother, Disana's father, had come to China and spent a week watching Disana slowly but surely slip away from the fragile hold of the life-support system.

"Have you done anything that could have exposed you to infection?" asked Disana's aunt. The question was curt and unsympathetic, perhaps even accusatory. She had not heard that question in more than ten years. She could not believe that anyone still asked that question.

"Well, well—it's just that I carried him to the car. I, I . . ." The American stuttered into silence.

"You don't get AIDS from carrying someone with a headache into a car," she sighed. Her phone rang.

"Have the Chinese changed their minds? Has the embassy been able to persuade them?" Disana's grandfather's voice was as clear as if he were in the next town. The time to worry about the phone bills would be later.

"The Chinese won't budge. They insist on a burial here or a cremation."

"Cremation is totally out of the question."

"I know, Dad."

"Your mother says you must try harder at convincing the Chinese."

"Dad, we must accept that we are going to have to bury him here."

The Chinese refused to give in, so Disana was buried in China. His funeral was the talk of the village, on account of having a service with no body and no coffin. His cause of death was never publicly stated. Everyone knew, but no one named it. His hospital records in Botswana, neatly handwritten by the same nurse who had first persuaded him to get tested, simply state: "lost to follow-up."

It seems sadly ironic that Disana would die of AIDS in China. The AIDS situation there is quite different from that in Botswana. Fewer than 1 in every 1,000 adults in China is infected with HIV, as opposed to 1 of 4 four adults in Botswana. And most of the Chinese who have gotten infected were exposed by illicit injection-drug use, not by sex, as in Botswana.

China has, however, had experience with other frightening epidemics of infectious diseases. In 2003 an epidemic of SARS, or severe acute respiratory syndrome, broke out in China and killed a large fraction of those who were infected. Like AIDS, it was a new viral disease. Unlike HIV/AIDS, it was easily spread by sneezing, coughing, or shaking unwashed hands. And unlike AIDS, it killed people soon after exposure, not years later. About a decade ago, another new infectious disease was reported as originating in China—bird flu. More lethal than other, earlier types of influenza, it too was spread by coughing and sneezing. These days, as you enter a major airport in China from outside the country, a monitor checks your body temperature. If you have a fever, you can't enter, at least not without a medical exam. This practice was started around the scares precipitated by SARS and bird flu, and it is still in place five years later for swine flu. Perhaps this helps explain why Chinese officials are so afraid of HIV, insisting on the isolation or cremation of a person who died of AIDS, even though the virus actually would pose no risk to those handling the body.

It is also surprising that Disana would die of cryptococcal meningitis just a few weeks after arriving in China. This happened two years after his wife died and a few months after her ex-boyfriend died, so they probably were infected earlier than Disana. It seems likely, though not certain, that Disana was infected by his wife.

Cryptococcal meningitis usually occurs at one of the final stages of HIV infection, when the CD4 lymphocyte count is very low and the patient is seriously debilitated with AIDS disease, and near death. In Disana's case it almost appears as if he was not on HAART therapy, or that the drugs were not working for some reason, even though he left Botswana with a four-month supply of medication. Once the meningitis was evident or a proper diagnosis was made, the immediate use of other antifungal drugs would have been necessary to save his life from this opportunistic infection.

The earlier stages of AIDS disease, usually seen when CD4 lymphocyte numbers have dropped to a third or a quarter of normal levels, include weight loss, chronic diarrhea, swollen lymph nodes, and the white pasty thrush in the mouth. Infections of the lungs, especially TB and some bacterial pneumonias, also occur, usually a bit later. As the HIV kills more and more immune cells and levels of CD4 cells fall to only 10 percent of normal or below, diseases such as cryptococcal meningitis, or TB that has moved beyond the lungs and throughout the body, often occur. At this stage, saving the patient is more difficult, but it can usually be done if both the HIV is treated (with HAART) and the meningitis is treated (with antifungal drugs like fluconazole). After AIDS patients have been on HAART for two to three years and the production of HIV in the body has been almost completely blocked, the immune system may recover to about half of the normal level of CD4 cells. Thus it seems surprising that Disana would leave for China at such an advanced stage of his immune suppression, when development of a final lethal opportunistic infection could occur. He was known to be confident and independent, and he seemed to retain these traits even as his body deteriorated. He did have signs and symptoms of confusion, depression, severe headaches, and deafness. These, along with fever, are typical with meningitis.

Disana left his three-year-old daughter with the grandparents. This is not unusual in Botswana, where the family unit is typically strong across generations, and the younger adults are more likely to work away from home. The supportive family structure also helps explain why orphanages are not very common, despite the large number of orphans. Placing a child in an orphanage is often construed as signaling a breakdown of the extended family, not just the death or debilitation of the child's parents. And children generally do better with family members than they do in orphanages. Disana's wife did undergo the preventive regimen of drugs during late pregnancy, so his daughter, who seems healthy at age three, is presumably uninfected. He also had his daughter retested and confirmed to be negative, just to be sure.

His wife originally hid the information about her HIV-positive status from Disana. To avoid detection, she also stopped taking the HAART drugs she had been on. This backfired, leading to a rapid recurrence of her disease and eventually death. She had apparently refused to resume taking the drugs. The reasons she stopped and failed to resume are probably complex, but interruptions in the drug regimen are not good. Depending on how long they last, the interruptions could rapidly result in the destruction of the new generations of immune cells associated with replacement and recovery. Guilt and depression about the likelihood of infecting her husband and others probably weighed in heavily, and the drugs can also have toxic side effects, which can cause people to stop taking them. The ways in which the drugs work against HIV are somewhat analogous to cancer chemotherapy, which often has serious side effects that are even more agonizing than those with ARVs. In fact, the drug AZT, one of the original ARVs that was regularly used to treat AIDS in Botswana, was first developed as a cancer drug. In 2008, AZT was replaced by Tenofovir as the drug of first choice for AIDS in Botswana. Tenofovir, developed more recently, causes fewer toxic side effects than AZT.

Drug resistance occurs more rapidly when interruptions occur. It can be a vicious cycle: the toxic side effects may lead to interruptions in taking the drugs; the interruptions may lead to drug resistance; and the drug resistance may lead to a need for new or different ARVs for treatment. The newer ARVs may be less toxic or have different side effects, but they are almost always more expensive, and in Africa, the cost of the drugs may be very important. The true cost of HIV/AIDS drugs may also be related to their propensity to cause toxic side effects and drug resistance. These factors lead to increased and more careful monitoring by experienced medical experts, and more lab tests. Such expenses may be much higher than the cost of the drugs alone, making the drugs more likely to be relatively unavailable in much of Africa.

At earlier stages of the epidemic, many thought that HAART would be inappropriate for use in Africa because of these limitations. Fortunately, we are now well beyond that general belief, and the use of ARVs in Africa has proven to be cost effective as well as morally appropriate. However, patients' adherence to or compliance with the drug regimen is of extreme importance, as is the organization of a medical-treatment system that results in the fewest people needing highly specialized care. The loss of Disana's wife and Disana was of ultimate importance to their immediate family, but they also represent an economic failure for the HAART treatment program. Their medical and drug expenses would have been offset by their return to society as functioning and productive workers and parents. When they lost their fight with AIDS, we all lost.

Disana, his wife, and his wife's ex-boyfriend all died at what seemed to be a relatively short time after their infection, and all three died at a time when HAART treatment was widely available in Botswana. Disana was started on drugs before he was visibly ill because his CD4 lymphocyte numbers were so low. This helps explain why he got a disease as severe as meningitis. Because all three died relatively soon after infection, we might wonder whether the HIV strain that was apparently common to all three was more rapidly lethal. This is possible, but the rapid course of their disease was more likely due to behavioral practices such as incomplete adherence to drug schedules, exposures to other germs, or just bad luck. However, research studies are under way in Botswana to try to sort out these kinds of questions. Some HIV-infected people develop AIDS within a year or two, while a few others appear to stay healthy for ten to fifteen years. This could be in part because some viruses replicate themselves more quickly or slowly, or it could be because some human genetic differences may help the body resist for longer periods of time.

In the end, Disana's hospital records in Botswana said "lost to follow-up." This is an expression often used in clinical therapeutic research trials when a study patient cannot be found. This can obviously happen when a patient has died. One can't help but wonder how often the final events are as sad and mysterious as they were for Disana, particularly in 2008, when the world has had experience with AIDS for more than twenty-five years.

Opelo's Rebellion

Issues of Adolescents and Women

OPELO, A SIXTEEN-YEAR-OLD girl-child was, physically, a beautiful human being and she knew it. She was also coming into womanhood, a bit early, it might be said, and was keen on asserting her independence. Although this was always going to pit her against her conservative parents, it was not in itself bad or unique. She could be moody and withdrawn. But she also seemed to want to take her clothes off, to show her beautiful self to the world. For her parents, she has been a nightmare. They have had to negotiate the lengthening of hems, which were receding alarmingly and threatening to turn her skirts into belts; the tightening of belts, to conceal underwear that was itself doing a bad job of hiding areas of her bottom that ought to remain private; the pulling up of flimsy garments that to them should be underwear, not outerwear.

Not only did Opelo rebel by wearing outrageously revealing clothing: when a local newspaper started "the Page 3 girls," she was among the girls queuing to take off their clothes for the coveted spot. While she did not make it into the newspaper, it is quite likely that someone somewhere has photographs of her that he whips out on occasion to titillate himself. The photographers involved were much older than their subjects. And then Opelo started drinking and perhaps smoking dope.

When negotiation failed to tame these impulses of their daughter's, to fling her beauty at the world in ways that were outright inappropriate, the parents resorted to begging, nagging, shouting, silences, and even beatings. Aunts and uncles were enlisted to talk sense into the young girl. Bribes were offered: a new cell phone, an expensive hairdo, a driving lesson . . .

"Opelo, child of my brother, what do you want?" an aunt asked in desperation at yet another meeting with her.

Nothing helped. Instead, things escalated; Opelo started sneaking out of the house on Friday nights, only coming back on Monday mornings—tired and apparently hungry, from the amount of food she ate—just in time to get ready for school. Midweek, she was like a caged animal, hissing at her siblings and eyeing her parents like they were her jailers. She whispered into her cell phone, which seemed to vibrate all the time, but would not say who her callers were.

"What makes it hard is how calmly and quietly she will look at you with those beautiful eyes! Never challenging you, never answering you back with disrespect! You think you have reached her and then the parents call to say she has not stopped!" one aunt lamented.

"Not challenging? No disrespect? I say that is exactly what she is doing by refusing to talk to anyone!" An older aunt had reached the end of her tether where Opelo was involved.

"At least she is still in school," the father sighed, thankful for small mercies.

"She is going to become pregnant, at this rate," the mother said, giving voice to what both were thinking.

At first, the biggest monster of them all, HIV, was not mentioned, but no doubt thoughts about that were ricocheting in their minds as well. After all, one of her aunts was herself nearly skeletal from the ravages of AIDS.

While the difficult teenager is a worldwide and age-old phenomenon, the nature of the challenges and dangers associated with that period of life will depend, to some extent, on what is available as a prohibited "pleasure" in a particular culture and time. Thankfully, though, in the majority of cases the phase passes, the child becomes an adult, and she no longer needs someone else to tell her that it is not in her interest to behave inappropriately. She might even have found a sport or some other interest to contain her boundless energy.

In the case of Opelo, the prohibited pleasures in her household were the standard ones, and they included not being home by 9:00 PM, smoking, drinking, sex, and disrespecting her elders.

Her mother was a member of the inner circle of a religious group that held all-night events during which members sang, danced, and clapped hands as the Holy Spirit possessed them and brought them closer to God. Her father was a respected member of his extended family, and he spoke authoritatively of family unity, respect for elders, and the importance of teaching the younger generation traditional values. Opelo's family was considered to have a home where there was *molao,* that is, family law and order—a family unlikely to raise a wayward child.

Because Opelo's rebellion took place as it did, in Botswana in the early years after 2000, it exposed her to various dangers, including HIV infection. When Opelo started missing school on Friday afternoons and Monday mornings and was observed being dropped off by different cars, the fear of HIV could not remain unvoiced anymore. It was clear that some older men were taking advantage of Opelo and she was engaging in what has now come to be termed, in HIV/AIDS-speak, "intergenerational sex."

"My daughter, these men just want sex from you! Nothing else, I swear to you!"

"My daughter, don't be fooled by the compliments about how beautiful you are. It is just to lure you into bed."

"That man must be at least thirty-five! He is as old as your uncle here. Can't you see what's happening? Aren't you afraid of HIV?"

"My daughter, these men are using you! They will spit you out like phlegm when they are done."

"Child of my brother, these are sugar daddies!"

Indeed they were sugar daddies, although Opelo could not have cost any one of them much; a cell phone, some spare cash, a pair of Nike shoes, a pair of sunglasses, lacy underwear—nothing her own parents were not willing to give her themselves, to get her out of the clutches of men they saw as the ruin of their daughter.

And they had plenty of examples around them, within their own extended family, of young girls whose high school education had been derailed by pregnancy. Pregnancy, illness, death . . . These were what they expected to be the fruits of what Opelo was sowing.

And hadn't she seen how her own aunts had died only a couple of years ago? Or how another aunt was blistering all over her body? Or how her own cousin was nursing a crippled and wheelchair-bound husband of only two years? How could she put herself in jeopardy in the face of all this evidence?

Opelo's father cannot bear to talk about her in public; it brings tears to his eyes. A simple day-to-day greeting of "How are the children? Are they well? How is Opelo?" is met by his averted eyes, a quick nod, and a change of subject.

Opelo's mother had a stroke that landed her in the hospital, and she nearly lost her job as a result. Since then, she has seemed absent-minded and she requires her husband's constant attention. No one openly blames Opelo for the stroke, but innuendos abound.

"Children of today, they can send you to an early grave," a relative utters.

"If your child will still answer you when you call, call yourself lucky," another responds.

Two years later though, mercifully, her father says Opelo is still in school—miraculously—and has not gotten pregnant. The high school leaving exams are just starting and Opelo seems to be taking her studying seriously. "If she can only write her final exams," her father prays, "then even if she falls pregnant, she can pick up later when she gets out of this cloud she is in!" Opelo's father never went to high school, and his dream is that all his three children will receive university educations. Opelo is his firstborn, and he was preparing her for this future by sending her to private school. Some members of the family blame private schools for the disintegration of family values. They argue that it is Western education that is eroding traditional values, resulting in wayward behavior all around.

"If she is on the pill, then she might have caught something worse than pregnancy!" Her mother voices the ever-present fear. "Let's hope she was using condoms! Let's just hope!"

"But you know that it is exactly because these men do not want to use condoms that they sleep with young girls! They want to protect themselves but do not want to use condoms. So they sleep with young girls!"

A conservative estimate puts the number of lovers Opelo had during the two-year period at five: all older men and all, from all accounts, married men. She has, over the past six months or so, started dressing "normally," but she does not seem to be able to get back to keeping the company of her peers, many of whom had ostracized her for "running around with married men." She still has an older man as a lover, but she has started to be involved more and more in family events. The two-year madness seems to be winding down to a close. Or is it?

✿

Girls or young women like Opelo are more likely to have sex with older men, as compared with young men having sex with older women. This results in age-related differences in infection rates with HIV. In the countries of southern Africa where HIV infection is so common, up to a third of young women may be infected by their early twenties. At the same age, perhaps only one in ten or one in twenty young men are infected. By age forty, more men are infected than women, as most of the women who got infected at an earlier age have already died. At least this was the situation before the widespread availability of antiretroviral drugs in Botswana, particularly the three-drug combination used for highly active antiretroviral therapy.

It has been reported that some HIV-infected men in Africa believe that having sex with a virgin girl will cure them of AIDS. But this is probably not a major reason why young women become infected with HIV in Botswana. A more likely scenario is that most men in the early stages of HIV infection do not know they are infected.

Understandably, women want to become pregnant to have children, and pregnancy and childbirth before marriage are common in Botswana. For about a decade we have been conducting clinical research trials in Botswana to test drugs and vaccines against HIV. We have also done research on other issues, such as how to identify early infections, how to slow down the rate of disease development, and how to identify genetic and other factors that increase the risk of infection. When we conduct these studies, two factors stand out. First, more women than men volunteer for the trials. This could be because more women than men are infected and ill with AIDS in the age groups that we consult. But it might also be that women feel a greater need to find additional ways to control their own destiny with respect to HIV/AIDS. The second factor that stands out is the higher than expected pregnancy rate among women who participate in the trials.

For research trials that test vaccines or drugs for the treatment of AIDS, women who volunteer are asked to state that they do not intend to get pregnant. But we found, for example, that about 20 percent of women who were ill with AIDS, and were successfully treated, became pregnant during a three-year trial. The women had been asked to refrain from getting pregnant in part because some of the drugs or vaccines being tested have been thoroughly tested only in men, and the possibility that they could cause fetal abnormalities or birth defects may not have been ruled out. Additionally, it seems important to strongly discourage pregnancy for HIV-positive women, whether in trials or not, to prevent the risk that more HIV-infected infants will be born. And in trials designed to prevent mother-to-child transmission of HIV in pregnant women, we have found that a significant number of women who have already participated in prevention trials, and received selected drugs to reduce maternal-infant transmission, reappear in the new trials with a subsequent pregnancy. This happens after careful counseling about the importance of not getting pregnant. The urge to procreate can be very strong.

In some situations, an HIV-negative woman has an HIV-positive partner or husband. "If she is on the pill, then she might have caught something worse than pregnancy," states Opelo's mother. "Let's hope she was using condoms." If an HIV-negative woman wants to have sex and avoid becoming infected herself, she and her partner can use condoms. However, if the woman wants to become pregnant, condoms cannot be used. Any barrier method that allows sperm to pass and survive will certainly also allow HIV to survive. To overcome this problem and allow women to have safe sex with a partner who is HIV-positive or of unknown HIV status, without a condom, research has been under way to develop microbicides.

Microbicides, to be used in the form of a vaginal lubricant or suppository, are substances that could kill any HIV that a woman is exposed to in semen. As such gels could be used without the knowledge of the partner, unlike a condom, this approach would be under the control of the woman. Unfortunately, the first generation of microbicides tested in women yielded disappointing results. They were designed as broad-spectrum disinfectants that would kill both HIV and other sexually transmitted infectious organisms, such as those that cause gonorrhea or herpes. But the experimental substances became diluted and were washed away after several hours, and they sometimes caused inflammation of the sensitive cells at the surface of the female reproductive organs. This approach backfired, making the women even more susceptible to HIV after the surface cells were damaged and the disinfectant had washed away. However, the next generation of vaginal microbicides looks more promising. Substances that cause inflammation are no longer being used, and antiretroviral drugs that are known to be selectively active against HIV have replaced the broad-spectrum disinfectants. In a few more years, we will know whether they are effective.

Opelo also started drinking and smoking dope. These activities obviously reduce inhibitions and make it more likely that one's behavior might result in risky sex. This could mean an increased chance of sex with partners whose HIV status is unknown, or an increased chance that condoms are not used. Either way, alcohol consumption increases risky sexual behavior and thereby increases the risk of HIV infection. Drinking seems to be a major contributor to the size of the epidemic in Botswana, whether it is *chibuku,* the homemade beer, or refined alcohol in the expensive bars and hotels. Smoking marijuana is also a problem in some regions of the country. The injection-drug use associated with major HIV epidemics in other parts of the world is rare in Botswana.

Sex—and pregnancy—is not unusual for teenage girls. Yet most new procedures for HIV-prevention are not generally tested in teenagers. For example, much progress has been made by testing drugs in late pregnancy to reduce the risk that infants are born HIV infected. In Botswana, such drug tests could not be done with HIV-positive pregnant teenagers unless researchers obtained permission from their parents. Because many teenagers did not want their parents to know they were HIV infected, they could not participate in the trials. This greatly increased the risk that their newborns would also be HIV infected.

Opelo's own aunts had died recently, presumably from HIV/AIDS. Another aunt was "blistering all over her body," perhaps owing to a condition known as seborrheic dermatitis, which may arise from a bacterial infection relatively early during HIV infection, or to *molluscum contagiosum,* a pox-virus infection that occurs in 10 to 20 percent of AIDS patients late in their disease. Her cousin was nursing a "crippled and wheelchair-bound" husband of only two years. His condition may or may not be due to HIV. The virus can cause neurological conditions, including ataxia, a lack of muscle control. At the terminal stages of HIV wasting, severe emaciation may leave no strength for walking.

Perhaps Opelo has been fortunate enough to escape infection with HIV for now, but unless she has been tested it is too early to know, as the associated diseases might not be apparent until five to ten years after the exposure.

Desperation for Pono

Orphans of HIV/AIDS

"JUDGE, THERE IS SOMEONE on the phone who wants to speak to you." My secretary's voice sounded agitated.

"Please take their name and telephone number and let them know that I will call back later."

"He is crying, Judge. He says he must speak to you now. It's a young man; perhaps a boy. I think you should take the call."

"Do you know what it is about?"

"No, but he sounds desperate."

"Okay, put him through."

I had hoped for a quiet afternoon as I finished a judgment that had been pending for a while.

"Are you Chief Justice Unity Dow?"

"No, I am not the chief justice. Do you wish to speak to the chief justice?"

"I want to speak to Chief Justice Unity Dow."

"Well, I am Judge Dow, but if you wish to speak to the chief justice, I can reroute your call." I was hoping to be able to get out of the call. I couldn't imagine how I would be able to help the desperate-sounding young man at the end of the line. If his purpose was to inquire about a case that was taking too long to resolve, the registrar was a better bet. If he wanted to complain about the system, then perhaps the chief justice was the appropriate person. I was not involved in administration, and I was concerned that talking to me would simply increase his desperation.

"Are you Chief Justice Unity Dow? I have seen your name in the papers. You help women and children. I wish I were dead! I feel like killing myself." The voice had become strangled; the young man was crying.

"Can you tell me what your problem is?"

"All I want is to go back to school. My mother is dead and no one will help me. I have been to see social workers and Child Line and the DC. No one will help me. I am going to kill myself. It is better I kill myself."

"Who am I speaking to?"

"Pono."

"How old are you?" I was playing for time while I thought of what to do.

"Eighteen. I don't know what to do any more. I tried to kill myself and they saved me. I wish they had not saved me. I don't know why they saved me if they can't help me. My mother is dead and my life is finished."

"Where are you calling from?"

"Gaborone. Chief Justice, I hate my life. I just hate it!"

"Listen, Pono. Why don't you come here to Lobatse so we can talk?"

"I don't have any money for the bus fare."

"Do you think you can get a loan of five pula for the fare? I will give you the money so you can pay it back." There was a moment's hesitation before he agreed.

. . .

Within two hours a lanky, sad-looking young man entered my office.

"Thank you for seeing me. I am desperate. I don't want to die, but what else can I do? I tried before. I poured petrol on myself and set myself alight, but they saved me. For what? Let me show you." Pono stood up and was about to yank off his T-shirt when I stopped him. There was no need to disillusion the young man by showing that I was not able to handle injuries and bad scars; after all, he had ridden in a hot bus for an hour with hope of strength and support at the other end.

"Tell me about your mother."

"My mother is dead. She suffered before she died. I am the oldest. I have two brothers and a sister."

"Your father?"

"My father . . . The father of my brothers and sisters deserted my mother when she became ill. He never treated me well even before. He always beat me, but my mother pretended not to see. But now he deserted all of us. He is gone; doesn't care. He was not my real father."

"Who do you live with?"

"I just want to go back to school. We live with our grandmother and great-grandmother. My grandmother sells *chibuku* alcohol from the yard, so there is no quiet moment at all. How can my sister study, when she is always selling alcohol? And the men are always touching her. I refuse to help with the alcohol. I go to church. My other brother is lucky because he is in boarding school."

"Did your mother die of AIDS?" I have learned to ask the question directly and have also learned that such directness is appreciated.

"Yes." The answer was a whisper.

There was some quiet before he continued, "Nobody talks about it. But it is obvious. That silence is killing me! We all saw her waste away and die, but we don't talk about it!"

At the end of our meeting, I took Pono to his home so I could meet his family. I parked my vehicle in front of a yard full of men, about fifteen in all, in different stages of drunkenness. The yard was littered with empty *chibuku* cartons.

I got out of the vehicle, obviously not dressed for an afternoon at a *chibuku* depot. Most of the men were watching me, and true to form, one of them announced, "Hey, you, woman, come here. I love you. I want to marry you."

"I love you too. I want to marry you. You want to set a date?"

The man looked confused. I was supposed to be embarrassed and offended. He decided I was not interesting anymore, so he went back to his drunken rocking to music that was playing only in his head.

Pono led me past the men and a woman he introduced as his aunt, who was selling the *chibuku,* to the door of the best of three sorry-looking structures in the yard. Inside the first room I found a woman in her late sixties sitting on the floor. She did not seem to be doing anything in particular. She seemed to be just sitting, staring at the filthy wall less than fours meters from her. She offered me a seat, and as I sat down on the only sofa in the room, a cloud of dust rose, causing me to cough. I considered standing up but knew that that would be very impolite. I thought of fleas and lice attaching themselves to my clothes, but decided that, having gone this far, I just had to take my chances and hope for the best. From the next room, the door to which was open, I could hear the groaning of a person in pain. When I looked around, I could see a bony leg sticking out from a tangle of old threadbare blankets.

"That is my mother. She is very old and ill." The speaker herself seemed old and ill.

"I came to talk to you about Pono. He came to see me."

"Pono wants things he cannot have. Where are we going to get money to send him to school? He just wants to go to church and read the Bible. Will the Bible buy him food?"

"Maybe I can help."

"Oh, my child, you will help?"

"What did Pono's mother die of?"

"She was sick for a long time my child."

"AIDS?"

"Oh, my child, we don't say it like that. But yes. She was sick for a long time. She suffered, that daughter of mine, she suffered."

"The father of the children? Where is he?"

"Do they ever stick around, my child? They only want the women when times are good. Yes. When she was healthy, he was like a perennial river here; never dry! Now? You cannot even get a whiff of his smell. He is gone. I am left with the children! How can I take care of them? My mother is sick and old. I sell *chibuku* and Pono refuses to help. He says he will not touch alcohol. He wants to read the Bible the whole day! God helps those who help themselves! You must talk to him."

I looked around and wondered where, exactly, in this cramped setting Pono's mother had spent her last days. The building we were in, although the most decent of the three on the property, was a two-room concrete-walled structure with a corrugated iron roof. It was dark and it stank like one would expect, from too many bodies sleeping in too small a place. The curtains were tattered and torn, and the original color of the walls was not discernible. The other two buildings were no more than shacks. Pono, his brother who was at home, and his sister, together with other children whose relationship to them was unclear, slept in one of the shacks. The other shack was the *chibuku* depot as well as a kitchen of sorts. In all, eleven people slept in the three rooms, each no more than nine square meters. Where were the children's clothes or books? An old cupboard was the only other piece of furniture in the room we were in. If there was so little in the most decent room, how could there be more in the shack where the children slept?

It was not difficult to understand why, if one saw no exit from such misery, a person might wish to kill himself. Having seen the conditions under which the children lived, I agreed to pay the tuition for Pono's computer course and to give him a monthly allowance of 200 pula.

Within months, though, my involvement in the lives of Pono and his siblings had deepened. First, I tried to get the children's father to contribute to their upkeep. I sent him the following letter:

> Dear Sir,
>
> First let me introduce myself and explain my involvement in this matter. First, do understand that it is not in my capacity as a judge that I am writing to you, but rather as a private individual concerned about the welfare of the three children named below. Pono came to me under very sad circumstances and I agreed to assist him with his schooling. He had lost his mother, was living under very poor conditions and had three younger siblings to worry about. Indeed I paid his tuition at a computer school and gave him an allowance for personal expenses. Since then, I have been involved, on and off, in assisting Pono and his siblings. This communication takes my involvement to another level.
>
> My information is essentially as follows. Pono is the oldest child of one Nkamo Modise, now deceased. Pono has three younger siblings, namely Kopano, Tumisang and Lebo. You are the father of the children. Since the death of Nkamo, in 1998, you have neglected your children. Your children live in a compound in which a total of 11 people live, under very cramped and poor conditions. The compound also serves as a

chibuku outlet, with the result that an average of ten men, in all stages of drunkenness, can be observed sitting within, walking about and/or staggering around the compound. *Chibuku* selling is Pono's grandmother's main source of income. Your children survive on the proceeds of the *chibuku* sales as well as on social welfare rations. They were registered as orphans after their mother's death and your disappearance. Your children need your support. You are gainfully employed and should be making a contribution to the maintenance of your children.

It seems obvious that the following must take place:

a. The children must be moved from their current residence. Not only is their current living condition not conducive to studying, there is a real danger that your daughter will end up being raped by some drunk.

b. You must pay maintenance for the children. As a police officer, you must earn enough to support your children.

c. The children must receive counseling to help them deal with the death of their mother as well as your abandoning them.

d. Pono must assume the critical role of guardian to his younger siblings.

I have offered the children a house, for free, to be available on the first of July 2002, at which they can try to re-build their lives as a family, with Pono providing the guardianship role. I will make arrangements for a social worker to visit the children and to provide counseling.

Your own contribution will be in monetary terms, and I believe the sum of 200 per child per month is reasonable.

This will give Pono the sum of P600 per month to clothe, feed, transport the children, as well as to provide them with water, electricity and medical care. Kindly call me so we can meet and finalize these arrangements. Should you refuse, neglect or fail to get in touch with me, your children, assisted by Pono, will engage Ms. Stella Nkwe, an attorney in Gaborone, to institute legal action against you. I have offered to pay the legal fees on their behalf, expecting to collect them from you at the conclusion of the case.

I also wrote to the Social and Community Development Office, explaining how I got involved:

Dear Madam,

This is to explain to you how I got involved with Pono and his siblings. Pono first came to me when he was at the end of his tether and contemplating suicide. I agreed to pay for his NIIT computer course and indeed I did. I came to know the following about him. He is the oldest child of one Nkamo Modise, now deceased. He has three younger siblings, namely Kopano, Tumisang and Lebo. Since the death of Nkamo, in 1998, the children have been in the care of their grandmother who resides at Lot 2093 New Canada. I have been at that place on several occasions and found it less than ideal for young children. The children live in a compound in which a total of 11 people live, under very cramped and poor conditions. The compound also serves as a *chíbuku* outlet, with the result that an average of ten men, in all stages of drunkenness, can be observed sitting within, walking about and/or staggering around the compound. *Chíbuku* selling is Pono's grandmother's main source of income and it would be unfair to assume a superior attitude about this. After all, the children survive on the proceeds of the *chibuku* sales and social welfare rations. They were registered as orphans after their mother's death.

After months of giving Pono a P200 allowance, it seemed to me that the best thing would be to remove the children from their current environment. Thus my offer of alternative accommodation. My hope is that at the new residence the two youngest children (doing Standard 7) will do better in school and that Pono will find a job. Kopano is doing his Form V and is, at least, a boarder.

I am happy to hear that your office can assist with water and electricity bills.

Thank you and please do not hesitate to call should you require any clarification about this matter.

I am enclosing a copy of Deed of Transfer evidencing my ownership of Lot 2112 as well as the Memorandum of Grant of Use detailing the terms of Pono and his siblings' occupation of Lot 2112.

Memorandum of Grant of Use

Entered into by and between
Unity Dow [the owner]
And
Pono Modise [the occupant]

Whereas the owner is the registered owner of Lot 2112, Gaborone;

And whereas the occupant and his three siblings, whose mother Nkamo Modise is now deceased, are in need of accommodation;

And whereas the owner has been assisting the occupant financially for the past year and half and considers that additional assistance is necessary;

And whereas the owner has discussed the matter with the occupant's grand mother and great-grand mother and has offered assistance to the occupant and his siblings;

And whereas such offer of assistance has been accepted;

Now Therefore It Is Agreed as Follows:

1. The owner grants the occupant and his siblings, namely Kopano, Tumisang and Lebo, the right to reside at Lot 2112, Gaborone from the 1st May 2002 to 30th April 2004.

2. The occupant will take occupation of Lot 2112 and thereat establish a family comprising himself as its manager and leader and his siblings.

3. The grant of use shall be free of charge and is solely motivated by the occupant's family situation, namely that he has lost his mother, he and his siblings are living under cramped conditions and he is of limited means.

4. The grant of use may be extended at the termination of the current grant. Such extension will depend on various factors, including the earning situation of the occupant, the schooling situation of the siblings, and the manner in which the occupant and his siblings have conducted themselves at the premises.

5. The occupant and his siblings may not invite or allow any other person or persons to reside at Lot 2112, whether for free or for rewards, without the written consent of the owner.

6. The occupant and his siblings may not use the property for any purposes other than a family residence.

7. The occupant and his siblings will keep the property in a tidy and clean manner.

8. The occupant will play the role of guardian of his siblings

and as such will manage all financial matters associated with life at Lot 2112.

9. The occupant will be liable for all water and electricity charges.
10. The owner will be liable for city council rates charges.

Four years on, Pono is still the "parent" to his siblings. The brother who comes immediately after him has one more year to go at university, and the other two siblings have two years to go before they finish high school. Their father proved to be totally uninterested in his children and has failed to provide for their support. Through government orphan programs, the children have been fed, have been provided with school uniforms and supplies, and have had their utilities at the house paid for.

Pono did not do well in his computer course, so he has found it hard to find a permanent job. He has worked at two different jobs in the past four years, and during and between those, he has been a stabilizer in the small family that he heads. The children are doing well in school and one of them will be graduating from university next year!

❖

Perhaps two million children in the world are infected with HIV, either by being born to an HIV-positive mother or by sexual transmission after they reached puberty. Most of those who were infected by their mothers are, or will become, orphans, at least in situations where the life of the mother was not saved by HAART treatment. In most situations, either the father initially infected the mother or the mother infected the father, so both parents are eventually lost to HIV/AIDS.

While about a third of the infants born to HIV-positive mothers become infected, the prophylactic use of antiretroviral drugs in late pregnancy reduces the number of infants infected. The most common intervention used to reduce infant infections from HIV-positive mothers is the administration of one dose of nevirapine, given to the mother at the time of delivery. This is effective in reducing the number of infected infants by about 50 percent. It is still the most common procedure used in Africa, where only about 10 percent of HIV-positive mothers receive anything at all to reduce the chance of infant infection. It is often judged to be the only option available when a pregnant woman is not discovered to be HIV positive until she presents for delivery. In the more typical situation in Botswana now, the pregnant woman is found to be HIV positive several months before delivery, and she can be put on drugs like AZT, or even HAART antiretroviral combinations, six to twelve weeks before delivery. This may reduce the rate of neonatal infections by 90 percent or more.

When nevirapine alone is given to the mother at delivery, she often develops resistance to the drug. If she is then treated soon after for her own disease with a HAART combination that includes nevirapine, or a related drug, the therapy may be ineffective. When AIDS therapy doesn't work, the mother dies and the child becomes an orphan, even though he or she has been protected from HIV. Because of research trials recently done in Botswana, we now know that short-course nevirapine should not be given to pregnant women.

Thus, although some AIDS orphans are themselves infected with HIV, most are not. Perhaps 15 million children in the world are AIDS orphans. Most are in Africa, and most in countries where the social systems are grossly inadequate. As in the case of Pono and his siblings, the extended family remains the predominant caregiving unit for the orphaned children, but it is rarely able to provide the support needed. It has been estimated by some that up to a third of all children in southern Africa might become AIDS orphans by 2010. In Botswana and Namibia, at least, the recent availability of HAART should prevent this dire situation. In the past six to eight years, since the increased use of drugs to reduce maternal transmission, the number of infants born with HIV has dropped. But the number of adult patients being treated with HAART for their AIDS disease has not expanded as rapidly. Until the pace of treatment catches up, there will be more orphans.

The lack of a support system, illustrated by Pono's situation when he contacted Judge Dow, is not unusual. Many households are large and headed by elderly grandparents or by the older children themselves. Quite a few include orphans from more than one family. Conditions of extreme poverty and crowding are common. Sex crimes, particularly against girls, increase in the absence of supervision and adult protection. Teenage girls in orphan situations are more likely to become commercial sex workers, out of desperation, and thus greatly increase their own risk for HIV infection. Formal education may be terminated or interrupted, and child labor practices increase. Psychological trauma may occur, as happened with Pono, who became suicidal. The stigma of being an orphan may cause even more stress than poverty or the situation of parental HIV illness.

Although orphaned due to AIDS, it seems likely that Pono and his siblings were born before their mother was infected, and thus were not at risk of direct infection themselves at the time of birth. However, Pono's situation provides a vivid example of how HIV affects many more than those who are directly infected. It also shows that siblings may have strong motivation to care for each other.

· 16 ·

Government Action Makes a Difference

A Nation Responds

BOTSWANA HAS OFTEN BEEN DESCRIBED as an African country that got it right—a stable democracy and an expanding economy with low rates of corruption. Much of the credit for this can be attributed to three great men—Sir Seretse Khama, who was president from 1966 to 1980, Sir Ketumile Masire, who was president from 1980 to 1998, and Festus Gontebonye Mogae, who was president from 1998 to 2008. Yet their success was also made possible by many of the citizen-leaders and members of Parliament who were willing to make sacrifices for the good of the country. The tribal leaders also used their power in constructive ways, through the House of Chiefs. Ironically, however, the nation's growing economy and general attitude of social acceptance may have contributed to the expansion of the HIV epidemic. Botswana had very few paved roads, few private vehicles, and a very modest system of public transportation in the 1970s. By the 1990s, improved conditions meant many young adults were frequently moving between positions of employment in Gaborone or Francistown and their home villages, often carrying HIV with them. A general guideline in Africa was that HIV rates were higher in the cities than in the rural villages. In Botswana, the rural villages were rapidly catching up.

The epidemic of HIV transmission began to expand in the late 1980s in most of southern Africa, and the epidemic of AIDS disease followed five to ten years later, allowing for the usual lag time before the immune system is destroyed in infected individuals. Peak rates of AIDS disease in Botswana and the rest of southern Africa occurred in 2000 to 2004, at least a decade after the peak in America and the rest of sub-Saharan Africa. A great surprise was that the rates of infection and disease were much higher in southern Africa. Was this because of different sexual practices, such as multiple concurrent relationships? Lower circumcision rates? A different virus? Different genetic backgrounds in the people? All of the above?

Botswana, Namibia, and the Republic of South Africa are three of the richest countries in Africa. Per capita income for these countries at the turn of the new millennium was almost up to that of Thailand and Brazil, countries that were often given high marks for the active governmental responses to their own AIDS epidemics, which occurred at about the same time, or slightly before, the epidemic hit Botswana. But HIV infection rates in southern Africa were twentyfold higher than in Brazil or Thailand. The cost of responding with drugs for prevention of maternal transmission or for treatment would represent a far greater economic burden if 25 percent of young adults were infected, as compared with the 1 to 2 percent in Thailand or Brazil.

As HIV rates were becoming frighteningly high in 1996, President Masire invited Dr. Essex and his colleagues at Harvard University to visit Botswana to help analyze the situation and offer advice. At the time, Botswana had no AIDS experts; Harvard had many. Samples of blood were collected from AIDS patients and those with early HIV infections. It was soon apparent that the subtype of

HIV in Botswana was HIV-1C, different from the viruses that caused earlier epidemics in other parts of Africa. The Botswana-Harvard Partnership was established in Gaborone. It soon became the largest AIDS research institute in Africa.

President Mogae, who served at the peak time of the epidemic, was a skillful leader who soon became an AIDS activist, at least as a governmental official. Soon after taking office, he promised that he would never give a speech in Botswana without mentioning the AIDS problem and he appeared to fulfill this promise. He was also an Oxford-trained economist and a former minister of finance. So when he made recommendations to mobilize resources to fight AIDS, it was assumed that he had considered the financial implications.

A major source of income for Botswana is diamonds. Debswana, the company that operates the mines, is a partnership between the government of Botswana and De Beers, the large multinational European company that operates in several countries in Africa. The employees of Debswana who had AIDS were the first in Botswana to receive the life-saving drugs. This sent a clear message that saving lives of trained miners would be worth the cost of the AIDS drugs. Those who worked in the diamond mines were also given extensive education about HIV and AIDS. As a result, their rate of infection, at least according to voluntary tests, was lower than that of other adults in Botswana. Meanwhile, the opposite was occurring in other countries. In the Republic of South Africa, those who worked in mines had higher infection rates than other adults.

After the screening of blood donors began in the late 1980s, biennial surveys were undertaken to obtain more accurate estimates of the number of people infected. Pregnant women were screened when they visited prenatal health care clinics. Men with sexually transmitted diseases were screened when they came in for care. The HIV testing was done anonymously. Later there would be door-to-door surveys. Centers for voluntary testing and counseling were also established, first in Gaborone, and then all over the country.

By 1999 or 2000, it became apparent that drugs such as AZT and nevirapine could be used to reduce the rate at which infected mothers infected their infants. By 2005 or 2006, the program to prevent mother-to-child transmission covered 80 to 90 percent of all Batswana mothers. The government program began giving the drugs earlier in gestation when it became apparent that this was even better. And it began giving HIV-positive mothers formula for their babies, to prevent infections through breastfeeding. It was already providing *tsabana,* a high-protein gruel, to young infants.

The government erected a building for the Botswana-Harvard Partnership that was opened on World AIDS Day in 2001. Located on the campus of the largest hospital in the country, it serves as a reference center for tests needed to diagnose and treat AIDS, for research, and for teaching. Other partners were encouraged to set up bases for their AIDS activities in Botswana. These included pediatricians from Baylor University and infectious disease experts from the University of Pennsylvania. The U.S. Centers for Disease Control and Prevention, which was already doing TB research in Botswana, expanded it work to include HIV/AIDS. The Gates and Merck foundations made substantial financial commitments through a new agency called the African Comprehensive HIV/AIDS Partnerships (ACHAP). The Secure the Future Foundation, an arm of Bristol-Myers Squibb, built a new AIDS center for children and financed treatment trials. The pharmaceutical companies Glaxo Wellcome, Boehringer Ingelheim, Merck, and Bristol-Myers Squibb all donated drugs for either research or general treatment, or both. The Clinton Foundation, the World Health Organization, and the Global Fund all got involved. PEPFAR, the U.S. President's Emergency Program for AIDS Relief, initiated by President Bush, selected Botswana as one of about fifteen countries to which it provided funds. If you wanted to determine how to save Africa from AIDS, Botswana was the place to be. Everyone wanted a piece of the action. President Mogae's strategy was paying off.

In late 2001 and early 2002, the Masa treatment program—"A New Dawn" in Setswana—was begun. The government made huge block purchases of a combination of three HAART drugs. At first the numerous severely ill patients were triaged, in an effort to save as many lives as possible. Those with TB and the parents of young children were given preference. Saving the parents would help alleviate the orphan problem; treating those AIDS patients who had TB would also reduce TB transmission generally, not just among people with HIV. The Masa program steadily expanded. Within several years, it had grown from four initial treatment sites—in Gaborone, Francistown, Maun, and Serowe—to about thirty-five sites throughout the country. Roughly 85 percent of those who needed HAART treatment were now on it, a percentage that was the envy of the rest of Africa, equivalent even to the countries in the developed world, which had far fewer patients to treat.

The expansion of treatment and prevention programs required the training of personnel. Physicians, nurses, pharmacists, counselors, and laboratory personnel who had experience with HIV/AIDS were rare in Botswana when the treatment program began. The KITSO training program—Knowledge, Innovation, and Training Shall Overcome AIDS (kitso also means knowledge in Setswana)—was organized by Harvard and the Ministry of Health, and funded by ACHAP. It began training medical staff, offering courses to more than 5,000 individuals within a few years. The program was linked to government certification of medical personnel for the prescription of AIDS drugs, assuring that the drugs would be used properly.

The governmental Masa program was already well established at the time PEPFAR funding began to arrive, reducing the need for assistance for direct care and treatment. But the country got permission to use the PEPFAR money for monitoring and evaluation, to verify that the quality of treatment was high. It turned out to be very high.

Research was conducted to determine which drugs worked best for treatment of adults and children and at what level of immune-cell deterioration to begin treatment in order to save the most lives and the most pula (the currency of Botswana). Research was also conducted on when to start drug therapy during pregnancy to prevent HIV transmission from mother to fetus, which drugs to use, and how best to reduce infant HIV infection and AIDS through drug prophylaxis while breastfeeding. And research was conducted in areas that might pay off only later—vaccine development, how drug-resistance variants develop and are transmitted, and which types of behavioral interventions, such as circumcision, work against HIV/AIDS. Even more basic research was endorsed, asking questions such as why the immune system was destroyed by the virus, and how the genetics of the virus and the genetics of people counterbalanced each other through evolution to produce virulence or protection.

Another initiative of President Mogae's was the "opt-out" program. Anyone who entered a state-sponsored health facility for any reason was asked if they wished to refuse an offered AIDS test. Most did not refuse the test. Initially criticized by some human rights advocates, the program produced the desired results: many more people were placed on treatment, and many more knew that they were infected. Those in the latter group could then be counseled closely to reduce the chances that they would infect others. They could also be monitored more closely for loss of CD4 immune cells, to make sure they received drug treatment before much damage could occur. Free treatment was offered to all who could not pay.

Many countries in Africa that had both an HIV problem and a tourism industry tried to cover up or pretend that AIDS was not a problem. Botswana is a major site for wildlife tourism but it took the opposite approach, revealing to the world that it was proactive about AIDS. It worked. The tourism industry expanded. The national police force and Debswana's employees often became eager participants in research projects. This was governmental leadership in action.

A few other countries in Africa have also mounted strong, constructive responses to their epidemics of HIV/AIDS. They, too, are unusual. Senegal, for example, started extensive education and condom-distribution programs at the earliest possible stages; it had high rates of male circumcision, related to religious or cultural practices; and commercial sex workers were licensed, and were required to have periodic HIV tests and health exams to keep their license. As a result, HIV prevalence rates never rose much above 1 percent in Senegal. Uganda also deserves much credit for being the first African country to begin treating AIDS patients with HAART regimens through a governmental program, beginning even before Botswana did. However, because of fiscal limitations the government often turned the patients over to private practitioners, which frequently led to problems with expertise and drug availability. A substantial number of the AIDS patients in Uganda have now been treated. The rates for treatment in Uganda are way above those of most African countries. But they are still way below Botswana's.

A disappointment is that, overall, prevalence rates have remained the same, or even increased, as more lives have been saved with drugs, and rates of new infections have not decreased as rapidly as had been hoped. Most prevention strategies, whether through vaccine development or changes in behavior, have been disappointing. But the success of drugs for the prevention of maternal transmission has been impressive. We at the Botswana-Harvard Partnership, and others, are now investigating the possibility that some of those same drugs can be used to prevent sexual transmission between adults.

The future of the AIDS epidemic is not certain, even in Botswana. The country has been surrounded by denialism about AIDS in South Africa and general governmental deterioration in Zimbabwe. Refugees and immigrants from all over southern Africa see Botswana as the place to be. This obviously increases tension, as well as demand on programs with limited resources. Treatment success also has its limitations. But Botswana has strong and consistent leadership at the top. It is hard not to be optimistic. Saturdays have been reclaimed!

Glossary

ACHAP African Comprehensive HIV/AIDS Partnerships. Established by the Bill and Melinda Gates Foundation and the Merck Foundation to provide support for AIDS education, treatment, and prevention in Botswana.

acute phase Early stage of infection with HIV. Occurs one to two months after initial infection. Often associated with flulike symptoms.

adeno 5a A genetically engineered version of a human virus that normally causes the common cold. The engineered version was designed to deliver selected genes of HIV in a harmless way, as a vaccine vector.

AIDS Acquired immune deficiency syndrome. Caused by HIV. Destruction of the immune system associated with opportunistic diseases such as tuberculosis and Kaposi's sarcoma.

AIDS-defining illness Disease, such as tuberculosis, cryptococcal meningitis, or Kaposi's sarcoma, that occurs at very high rates in patients with HIV/AIDS.

AIDS-risk genes   Human genes that increase or decrease the risk for infection with HIV, the rate of AIDS disease progression after infection with HIV, or both.

Alluvia   A heat-stable version of the drug Kaletra (also called lopinavir/ritonavir), designed so that it does not require refrigeration and can be used more readily in developing countries.

antibodies   Complex protein molecules made by the body in response to infection.

antibody tests   Laboratory tests designed to identify or diagnose an infection based on the antibodies induced.

antifungal drugs   Drugs designed to attack fungal diseases such as oral thrush caused by *Candida* or meningitis caused by *Cryptococcus,* both of which are common opportunistic infections in AIDS patients.

ARVs   Antiretrovirals. Drugs designed to stop HIV, a retrovirus, from replicating in the body.

ataxia   Inability to coordinate muscle movement.

Atripla   A three-drug combination of efavirenz, emtricitabine, and tenofovir (ARVs) mixed together in the same pill.

AZT   Zidovudine. Also called ZDV. The first ARV discovered. Still widely used.

Boehringer Ingelheim   Drug company that makes the ARV nevirapine.

bone marrow   The pasty material inside bones that represents the source of new cells to seed the blood. Provides progenitors of both red blood cells, or erythrocytes, for oxygenation, and white blood cells, such as lymphocytes and neutrophils, to fight infections.

Bristol-Myers Squibb (BMS)   Large pharmaceutical company that makes several ARV drugs.

cachexia   A state of generalized weakness and weight loss due to a progressive chronic disease state such as occurs with AIDS or cancer.

Candida albicans   A yeastlike fungus that often infects AIDS patients and causes oral thrush.

CD4   The primary receptor on immune cells to which HIV attaches, which allows infection to occur.

CD4 *cells*   The subset of immune cells that contain CD4 receptors, thus making such cells a primary target for HIV infection.

CD4 *count*   A calculation of the number of CD4-containing lymphocytes in blood. The CD4 count decreases as HIV kills cells and AIDS develops.

cervical cancer   Cancer of the uterine cervix.

chemoprophylaxis   The use of chemotherapeutics (drugs) to prevent infection with HIV. Often carried out by giving ARVs to pregnant women and infants to prevent the maternal HIV from infecting the infant during pregnancy, birth, or breastfeeding.

chimeric progeny viruses   Hybrid viruses produced when a patient gets infected with two different HIVs that are distinct from each other.

chromosomes   Elongated pieces of DNA in cells made by stringing together many genes.

chromosomal DNA   Pieces of DNA in a chromosome. May include the genes of HIV when the virus copies its RNA into DNA and the DNA integrates into chromosomes, as routinely occurs with HIV infection when the virus replicates itself in the body.

circumcision   A surgical procedure to remove the foreskin of the penis.

Combivir   An ARV treatment against HIV that combines zidovudine and lamivudine (3TC) in the same pill.

coreceptor   A molecule at the surface of susceptible cells that combines with CD4 to allow HIV to attack and penetrate. CCR5 and CXCR4 are designators for the coreceptors most commonly used by HIV.

Cryptococcus neoformans   A yeastlike fungus that often causes infections in the brains of advanced-stage AIDS patients.

cytolytic T cell vaccine   A type of experimental vaccine designed to stimulate immune cells that will kill infected cells directly rather than by making antibodies to mediate the immune attack.

DDI   Didanosine. A nucleoside analog reverse transcriptase inhibitor drug used against HIV. Also called Videx.

dementia   Loss of intellectual functions such as memory.

denialism   Movement by small group of people interested in AIDS who propose that HIV is actually not the cause of AIDS.

d4T   Nucleoside analog drug used against HIV; related to AZT. Also called stavudine, or Zerit.

didanosine   See DDI.

DNA vaccine   Experimental vaccine made with a naked strand of bioengineered DNA that directs the cells of the vaccinated person to make the relevant protein pieces, which in turn stimulate the immune response.

DOT   Directly observed therapy. A strategy for assisting patients to take their drugs on schedule by having a designated friend or family member assume responsibility for ensuring each drug dose is taken.

drug-resistant HIV   A mutant form of HIV able to replicate in the presence of selected drugs used to treat AIDS.

drug toxicity   Degree to which certain drugs have side effects associated with taking them, such as nausea, vomiting, or numbness of limbs.

efavirenz   A nonnucleoside reverse transcriptase inhibitor drug commonly used against HIV. Also called Sustiva or EFV.

efficacy trial   A research study conducted in a population of people. Usually randomized to determine whether a drug or vaccine shows a clinical benefit as compared with a placebo or a different drug.

emtricitabine   A nucleoside analog reverse transcriptase inhibitor drug used against HIV. Also called Emtriva or FTC.

false negative   A diagnostic test result (for HIV, in this case) that scores as negative when the person is actually infected. Because most HIV tests are based on production of antibodies, a false-negative test result for HIV may occur shortly after infection, before the body has had time to make the antibodies.

false positive   A diagnostic test result (for HIV, in this case) that scores as positive when the person is actually not infected. Because most HIV tests are based on production of antibodies, a false-positive test result for HIV may occur when the person acquired or developed antibodies without actually being infected with HIV. This can happen, for example, when an infant born to an HIV-positive mother receives her antibodies without receiving her virus, or when someone received an experimental HIV vaccine.

first-, second-, third-line therapy   First, second, and third combinations of antiretroviral drugs used to treat AIDS patients. The second-line therapy is used when, or if, the first line fails due to toxicity or drug resistance; third-line therapy is used if second-line therapy also fails.

FTC   See emtricitabine.

fungal encephalitis   Inflammation of the brain due to infection with pathogenic fungi, as may occur in AIDS patients.

generic drug   Drug made by secondary pharmaceutical company other than the company that first identified and patented the drug. Generic drugs are usually less expensive because the manufacturers do not incur the research and discovery costs needed to create the drugs.

gene sequence analysis   A laboratory procedure to decode the letters of HIV or HIV genes—for example, to determine how closely one

HIV is related to another or whether changes are present that may be related to drug resistance.

genetic code of HIV   The letter sequence of the virus; composed of about 10,000 nucleotide molecules.

genetic engineering   Use of biochemical techniques to design and synthesize genes or pieces of genes to make more efficient proteins or vaccines.

genetic variation   The extent to which one gene sequence is different from another (in this case, differences between HIVs).

genome   A complete copy of all the genetic information for an organism (in this case, HIV).

GlaxoSmithKline   Large pharmaceutical company that first introduced drugs AZT and 3TC, as well as Combivir, a pill that contains both.

Global Fund   The Global Fund to Fight AIDS, Tuberculosis and Malaria, a large multinational fund created to provide developing countries with resources to control those three diseases.

goiter   An enlarged thyroid gland.

gonorrhea   An infectious disease of the reproductive organs caused by the bacterium *Neisseria gonorrhoeae.*

gp120   Glycoprotein of 120,000 daltons in size that projects out from the surface of HIV. Frequent component of experimental vaccines and regularly used for diagnostic antibody tests.

HAART   Highly active antiretroviral therapy. A combination of antiretroviral drugs, usually three, that works effectively in AIDS patients to lower levels of replicating HIV to a minimal amount, allowing immune-cell production to recover. Virus is never completely eliminated and returns to elevated destructive levels if drugs are discontinued or drug resistance develops.

hairy leukoplakia   A raised white lesion on the tongue or mouth caused by the Epstein-Barr virus. AIDS patients have an elevated risk of developing such lesions.

hemophiliac   A person with a genetic disorder characterized by reduced ability of blood to coagulate. At the start of the AIDS epidemic, hemophiliacs had very high rates of HIV infections because they received transfusions of blood or blood-clotting factors from large pools of donors giving unscreened blood.

hepatitis B virus   A blood-borne virus that causes severe liver disease, sometimes progressing to liver cancer.

herpesvirus   A genus of large viruses that includes herpes simplex 2, a sexually transmitted virus that causes genital ulcers, and herpes simplex 1, a virus transmitted by mouth that causes lip ulcers and occasionally blindness in advanced-stage AIDS.

HIV   Human immunodeficiency virus.

HIV-1C   Subtype or clade of HIV-1 that constitutes a particular evolutionary branch. HIV-1C is dominant in southern Africa.

HIV proteins   Structural and enzymatic pieces of HIV viruses that provide shape, protection, and enzymatic functions for virus.

human papillomavirus   Virus that causes warts, including genital warts, and may cause cervical cancer.

incubation period   Time interval between initial infection and development of signs and symptoms of disease. Also called induction period.

immune evasion   Situation in which an infectious agent, such as HIV, can avoid attack and elimination by the immune system.

immune system   Dispersed collection of cells and molecules within the body that attack infectious agents and foreign substances.

incidence   Rate of new infections per year in a defined population, such as a city or country.

integration In the case of HIV, the process by which the DNA proviral stage of the virus inserts itself into the chromosomal DNA of the host cell.

IUD Intrauterine device. Inserted into uterus to prevent pregnancy, as means of birth control.

Kaletra Drug used to block replication of HIV by inhibiting the protease enzyme of the virus. Also called lopinavir/ritonavir, or Alluvia if in heat-resistant form.

Kaposi's sarcoma A form of cancer often associated with a purple discoloration on the skin or in the mouth. Occurs at high rates in people with immunosuppression.

KITSO Knowledge, Innovation, and Training Shall Overcome AIDS, a training program for health workers in Botswana on treatment and prevention of HIV/AIDS. *Kitso* is also the Setswana word for "knowledge."

lactic acidosis A metabolic disturbance due to accumulation of lactic acid, occurs as an occasional toxic effect associated with some AIDS drugs.

Langerhans cells Specialized form of immune cell occurring in skin and mucosal tissues, such as foreskin of penis. Langerhans cells are susceptible to infection with HIV.

laparoscopy Surgical procedure involving the insertion of an optical tube to examine organs in abdominal cavity.

latent A state of silent HIV survival in which the virus maintains its genome in infected cells without production of progeny virus. Later activation leads to virus production, cell killing, and disease.

lopinavir/ritonavir Drug designed to attack HIV by inactivating the viral protease enzyme. Boosted formulation of drug, also called Kaletra, or Alluvia if formulated to resist heat.

lymphadenopathy   Generalized swelling of lymph nodes or lymph "glands" due to infection of associated lymphocytes with HIV.

lymphocytes   Immune cells in blood and lymph nodes. A subset of lymphocytes called T4 or CD4 are particularly susceptible to infection and destruction by HIV.

lymphoma   A form of malignancy or leukemia associated with development of a tumorous mass of lymphocytes.

macrophage   Specialized immune cell that engulfs and processes foreign materials, including viruses. Provides specialized presentation of foreign material to lymphocytes that elicit specific immune reactions.

Masa   The national program to provide ARV treatment for HIV/AIDS in Botswana. Literally, "a new dawn" in the Setswana language.

MDR TB   Multi-drug-resistant strain of tuberculosis bacterium that grows in presence of major drugs used to treat TB.

meninges   Membranous sheath inside the skull that covers and protects the brain.

meningitis   Inflammation of meninges. Often caused by infection with fungus *Cryptococcus neoformans*.

Merck   Large pharmaceutical company that makes certain ARVs. Foundation partnered with Gates Foundation to establish ACHAP in Botswana.

microbicides   Experimental substances, to be used in vaginal suppository form, designed to kill HIV that may be in semen deposited during copulation.

mitochondrial toxicities   Toxic side effects associated with some ARVs, due to damage of cell mitochondria. Manifested as diverse symptoms, including muscle weakness.

molluscum contagiosum Disease of the skin caused by transmissible pox-type virus.

mopati A designated friend or family member of an AIDS patient charged with assuring that ARVs are taken on schedule by the patient.

mucous membranes Moist surface tissues at body sites such as vagina or inner foreskin of uncircumcised penis.

Mycobacterium tuberculosis Bacterium that causes TB.

nevirapine Also called NVP. An ARV that blocks HIV reverse transcriptase, but does so by a different mechanism from that used by nucleoside analog drugs such as AZT.

NVP See nevirapine.

obligative intracellular parasite Infectious agent, such as a virus, that can proliferate only after infecting living cells.

opportunistic infection Infectious disease, such as tuberculosis or cryptococcal meningitis, that occurs in immunosuppressed patient.

pancreatitis Inflammation of pancreas; may occur as a serious toxic side effect of certain AIDS drugs.

PCR Polymerase chain reaction, a technique to amplify genes. In this case, used to diagnose HIV infection in infants and to amplify amount of HIV in patients.

PEPFAR U.S. President's Emergency Program for AIDS Relief. Established by President George W. Bush to provide AIDS treatment and prevention in selected developing countries, especially in Africa.

peripheral neuropathies Pathology of nerves in arms or legs that may cause pain or numbness; may occur as toxic side effect with some AIDS drugs.

phase I, II, III trials Randomized, controlled trials for vaccines or drugs to evaluate toxicity and dosing levels in small numbers of volunteers (phase I), biological evidence of effect and safety in intermediate numbers (phase II), efficacy and expanded toxicity in larger populations of volunteers (phase III).

placebo Harmless, inert substance designed to appear indistinguishable from experimental vaccine or drug. Used in clinical trials as a control, to compare validity of toxic or efficacious effects of vaccine or drug.

plasma Liquid portion remaining after cells have been separated from whole blood.

polymerase chain reaction See PCR.

postexposure prophylaxis The use of HAART drugs to prevent the establishment of HIV infection when unintended exposures occur, such as for a health worker who has had an accidental needle stick involving blood from an HIV-positive person, or a rape victim in a region of high HIV prevalence.

prevalence Total rate of infection or disease. In this case, HIV prevalence is the fraction of the population infected, as defined by categories such as age, sex, or geographical location.

prophylactic drugs Antiretroviral drugs used to prevent the transmission of HIV, for example by HIV-positive mothers to their infants.

protease An enzyme that digests proteins in a particular way. HIV has its own specific protease that is needed for infection; this led to the development of drugs against HIV that are classified as protease inhibitors.

protective antibodies Those immune antibody molecules that attach to a virus (or other infectious agent) in such a manner that they block infection.

protozoa Single-cell infectious organisms unrelated to bacteria or viruses, such as malaria, that may cause disease. Some, such as the

Toxoplasma species, cause higher disease rates in people with HIV/AIDS.

pulmonary system   Tubes, such as trachea and bronchi, combined with lungs that process oxygen for the body. Serious infectious pneumonias are common in people who have AIDS.

recombination   Process by which microbes or viruses (in this case, HIV) can exchange genes to become chimeras with respect to their origin from different parental HIVs that caused a coinfection.

retrovirus   A virus of the family *Retroviridae,* such as HIV, that replicates by copying the viral RNA into DNA.

reverse transcriptase   The enzyme unique to HIV and other retroviruses that allows the virus to copy viral RNA into a DNA provirus, which is then integrated into chromosomal cellular DNA.

rubella   A viral disease characterized by skin lesions; also called German measles.

SARS   Severe acute respiratory syndrome. A highly lethal and highly contagious pneumonia first identified in China within the past decade. Caused by a coronavirus recently introduced to people from animals.

seborrheic dermatitis   A scaly skin eruption, usually on the face or scalp.

Secure the Future Foundation   Fund established by Bristol-Myers Squibb to provide resources for control of HIV/AIDS in selected African countries.

set point   Low point for viral load (VL) or minimal HIV replication that occurs after acute infection and before progression related to clinical AIDS symptoms.

slim disease   Form of clinical AIDS seen in Africa. Characterized by major weight loss.

stavudine   Anti-HIV drug, also known as Zerit and d4T, that functions as nucleoside analog reverse transcriptase inhibitor.

surveillance   Strategic monitoring of rates of HIV infection and/or development of AIDS disease.

Tebelopele   Network of government-supported centers for the voluntary testing and counseling of people who wish to determine their HIV status; located throughout Botswana.

tenofovir   Anti-HIV drug, also called Viread and TNF, that functions as a nucleotide analog to inhibit reverse transcriptase enzyme.

T4 cells   The same as CD4 cells. The subset of immune lymphocytes that are targeted during HIV infection.

3TC   Lamivudine, or Epivir. ARV used to inhibit HIV by functioning as nucleoside analog reverse transcriptase inhibitor.

thrush   White, yeastlike infection of the mouth with *Candida albicans*.

TNF   See tenofovir.

Trizivir   Tablet of ARV medicine that includes the three drugs abacavir, lamivudine, and zidovudine.

Truvada   Tablet of ARV medicine that includes tenofovir and emtricitabine in the same pill.

tsabana   Gruel-type food for infants that has high protein content.

Valium   Drug with generic name diazepam, used to reduce anxiety.

viral gene sequence   Genetic code of virus, in this case HIV. Used to determine degree of evolutionary relationship between different HIVs.

viral load (VL)   A quantitative measure of the amount of HIV in the blood. Used to determine the stage and severity of the infection and whether drug treatment is working.

virulence   The degree of disease-causing ability associated with a particular strain or category of infectious agent, such as HIV.

window period   Time after initial infection with HIV before antibodies are detectable. A concern for safe blood transfusions, as blood taken from an HIV-infected donor during this time may show a false-negative test result.

World Health Organization   International agency of United Nations charged with monitoring global rates of disease and making recommendations for good health practices and the prevention and treatment of diseases.

XTB   Extremely resistant strain of tuberculosis bacterium that grows in the presence of almost all of the drugs that can be used to treat TB.

ZDV   See zidovudine.

zidovudine   ARV drug that inhibits reverse transcriptase of HIV by functioning as nucleoside analog. Same as ZDV and AZT.

Further Reading

Chapter 1: The Epidemic

Chin, James. *The AIDS Pandemic: The Collision of Epidemiology with Political Correctness.* Oxford: Radcliffe, 2007.

Essex, Max, Souleymane Mboup, Phyllis J. Kanki, Richard G. Marlink, and Sheila D. Tlou, eds. *AIDS in Africa,* 2nd ed. New York: Kluwer Academic/Plenum, 2002.

Mboup, Souleymane, Rosemary Musonda, F. Mhalu, and Max Essex. "HIV/AIDS." In *Disease and Mortality in Sub-Saharan Africa,* 2nd ed., ed. Dean T. Jamison, Richard G. Feachem, Malegapuru W. Makgoba, Eduard R. Bos, Florence K. Baingana, Karen J. Hofman, and Khama O. Rogo, pp. 237–246. Washington, D.C.: World Bank, 2006.

UNAIDS. *2008 Report on the Global AIDS Epidemic,* Annex 1: *HIV and AIDS Estimates and Data, 2007 and 2001.* Geneva: UNAIDS, 2008. Available online at: http://data.unaids.org/pub/GlobalReport/2008/jc1510_2008_global_report_pp211_234_en.pdf.

Chapter 2: Sexual Transmission

Baeten, Jared M., and Julie Overbaugh. "Measuring the Infectiousness of Persons with HIV-1: Opportunities for Preventing Sexual HIV-1 Transmission." *Current HIV Research* 21 (2003): 69–89.

Balzarini, Jan, and Lut Van Damme. "Microbicide Drug Candidates to Prevent HIV Infection." *Lancet* 369 (2007): 787–797.

Beyrer, Chris. "HIV Epidemiology Update and Transmission Factors: Risks and Risk Contexts: 16th International AIDS Conference Epidemiology Plenary." *Clinical Infectious Diseases* 44 (2007): 981–987.

Wawer, Maria J., Ronald H. Gray, Nelson K. Sewankambo, David Serwadda, Xianbin Li, Oliver Laeyendecker, Noah Kiwanuka, Godfrey Kigozi, Mohammed Kiddugavu, Thomas Lutalo, Fred Nalugoda, Fred Wabwire-Mangen, Mary P. Meehan, and Thomas C. Quinn. "Rates of HIV-1 Transmission per Coital Act, by Stage of HIV-1 Infection, in Rakai, Uganda." *Journal of Infectious Diseases* 191 (2005): 1403–1409.

Wira, Charles R., and John V. Fahey. "A New Strategy to Understand How HIV Infects Women: Identification of a Window of Vulnerability during the Menstrual Cycle." *AIDS* 22 (2008): 1909–1917.

Chapter 3: Mother-to-Child Transmission

Breastfeeding and HIV International Transmission Study Group. "Late Postnatal Transmission of HIV-1 in Breast-Fed Children: An Individual Patient Data Meta-Analysis." *Journal of Infectious Diseases* 189 (2004): 2154–2166.

Chigwedere, Pride, George R. Seage III, Tun-Hou Lee, and Max Essex. "Efficacy of Antiretroviral Drugs in Reducing Mother to Child Transmission of HIV in Africa: A Meta-Analysis of Published Clinical Trials." *AIDS Research and Human Retroviruses* 24 (2008): 827–837.

Coovadia, Hoosen M., and Anna Coutsoudis. "HIV, Infant Feeding, and Survival: Old Wine in New Bottles, but Brimming with Promise." *AIDS* 21 (2007): 1837–1840.

Kumwenda, Newton I., Donald R. Hoover, Lynne M. Mofenson, Michael C. Thigpen, George Kafulafula, Qing Li, Linda Mipando, Kondwani Nkanaunena, Tsedal Mebrahtu, Marc Bulterys, Mary

Glenn Fowler, and Taha E. Taha. "Extended Antiretroviral Prophylaxis to Reduce Breast-Milk HIV-1 Transmission." *New England Journal of Medicine* 359 (2008): 119–129.

Montano, Monty, Matthew Russell, Peter Gilbert, Ibou Thior, Shahin Lockman, Roger Shapiro, Su-Yuan Chang, Tun Hou Lee, and Max Essex. "Comparative Prediction of Perinatal Human Immunodeficiency Virus Type 1 Transmission, Using Multiple Viral Load Markers." *Journal of Infectious Diseases* 188 (2003): 406–413.

Chapter 4: Diagnosis of HIV Infection

Constantine, Niel T., Guido van der Groen, Elizabeth M. Belsey, and Hiko Tamashiro. "Sensitivity of HIV-Antibody Assays Determined by Seroconversion Panels." *AIDS* 8 (1994): 1715–1720.

Creek, Tracy L., Raphael Ntumy, Khumo Seipone, Monica Smith, Mpho Mogodi, Molly Smit, Keitumetse Legwaila, Iris Molokwane, Goitebetswe Tebele, Loeto Mazhani, Nathan Shaffer, and Peter H. Kilmarx. "Successful Introduction of Routine Opt-Out HIV Testing in Antenatal Care in Botswana." *Journal of Acquired Immune Deficiency Syndrome* 45 (2007): 102–107.

Mine, Madisa, Keabetswe Bedi, Talkmore Maruta, Dignity Madziva, Modiri Tau, Tatenda Zana, Tendani Gaolathe, Sikhulile Moyo, Khumo Seipone, Ndwapi Ndwapi, Max Essex, and Richard Marlink. "Quantitation of Human Immunodeficiency Virus Type 1 Viral Load in Plasma Using Reverse Transcriptase Activity Assay at a District Hospital Laboratory in Botswana: A Decentralization Pilot Study." *Journal of Virological Methods* 159 (2009): 93–97.

Wright, Alexi A., and Ingrid T. Katz. "Home Testing for HIV." *New England Journal of Medicine* 354 (2006): 437–440.

Chapter 5: AIDS Disease in Adults and Availability of Treatment

All-Party Parliamentary Group (AAPG) on AIDS. *The Treatment Timebomb: Report of the Inquiry of the All-Party Parliamentary Group on AIDS into Long-Term Access to HIV Medicines in the Developing World.* London: APPG on AIDS, 2009. Available online at: http://www.aidsportal.org/repos/APPGTimebomb091.pdf.

Bussmann, Hermann, C. William Wester, Ndwapi Ndwapi, Nicolas Grundmann, Tendani Gaolathe, John Puvimanasinghe, Ava Avalos, Madisa Mine, Khumo Seipone, Max Essex, Victor deGruttola, and Richard G. Marlink. "Five-Year Outcomes of Initial Patients Treated in Botswana's National Antiretroviral Treatment Program." *AIDS* 22 (2008): 2303–2311.

Essex, Max, and Yichen Lu. "HIV/AIDS: Lessons from a New Disease Pandemic." In *Emerging Infections in Asia,* ed. Yichen Lu, Max Essex, and Bryan Roberts, pp. 133–142. New York: Springer, 2008.

Stevenson, Mario. "Twenty-five Years Later: Can HIV Be Cured?" *Scientific American* 299 (November 2008): 78–83.

Wainberg, Mark A. "Generic HIV Drugs: Enlightened Policy for Global Health." *New England Journal of Medicine* 352 (2005): 747–750.

Chapter 6: AIDS in Children

Coovadia, H. M., and Jane G. Schaller. "HIV/AIDS in Children: A Disaster in the Making." *Lancet* 372 (2008): 271–273.

Ioannidis, John P. A., Athina Tatsioni, Elaine J. Abrams, Marc Bulterys, Robert W. Coombs, James J. Goedert, Bette T. Korber, Marie Jeanne Mayaux, Lynne M. Mofenson, Jack Moye, Jr., Marie-Louise Newell, David E. Shapiro, Jean Paul Teglas, Bruce Thompson, and Jeffrey Wiener. "Maternal Viral Load and Rate of Disease Progression among Vertically HIV-1-Infected Children: An International Meta-Analysis." *AIDS* 18 (2004): 99–108.

Luzuriaga, Katherine, Margaret McManus, Lynne Mofenson, Paula Britto, Bobbie Graham, and John L. Sullivan, for the PACTG 356 Investigators. "A Trial of Three Antiretroviral Regimens in HIV-1-Infected Children." *New England Journal of Medicine* 350 (2004): 2471–2480.

Newell, Marie-Louise, Heena Brahmbhatt, and Peter D. Ghys. "Child Mortality and HIV Infection in Africa: A Review." *AIDS* 18, Suppl. 2 (2004): S27–S34.

Chapter 7: HIV and Tuberculosis

Chaisson, Richard E., and Neil A. Martinson. "Tuberculosis in Africa: Combatting an HIV-Driven Crisis." *New England Journal of Medicine* 358 (2008): 1089–1092.

Cohen, Gary M. "Access to Diagnostics in Support of HIV/AIDS and Tuberculosis Treatment in Developing Countries." *AIDS* Suppl. 4 (2007): S81–87.

Karim, Salim S. Abdool, Quarraisha Abdool Karim, Gerald Friedland, Umesh Lalloo, and Wafaa M. El Sadr, on behalf of the START Project. "Implementing Antiretroviral Therapy in Resource-Constrained Settings: Opportunities and Challenges in Integrating HIV and Tuberculosis Care." *AIDS* 18 (2004): 975–979.

Koenig, Robert. "Drug-Resistant Tuberculosis: In South Africa, XDR TB and HIV Prove a Deadly Combination." *Science* 319 (2008): 894–897.

Maartens, Gary, and Robert J Wilkinson. "Tuberculosis." *Lancet* 370 (2007): 2030–2043.

Chapter 8: Toxicities and Resistance to Drugs Used to Treat HIV/AIDS

Bisson, Greg, Robert Gross, Veronica Miller, Ian Weller, and Alexander Walker, on behalf of the Writing Group. "Monitoring of Long-Term Toxicities of HIV Treatments: An International Perspective." *AIDS* 17 (2003): 2407–2417.

Carr, Andrew, and Janaki Amin. "Efficacy and Tolerability of Initial Antiretroviral Therapy: A Systematic Review." *AIDS* 23 (2009): 343–353.

Clavel, François, and Allan J. Hance. "HIV Drug Resistance." *New England Journal of Medicine* 350 (2004): 1023–1035.

Johnson, Victoria A., Françoise Brun-Vézinet, Bonaventura Clotet, Huldrych F. Günthard, Daniel R. Kuritzkes, Deenan Pillay, Jonathan M. Schapiro, and Douglas D. Richman. "Update of the Drug Resistance Mutations in HIV-1: Spring 2008." *Topics in HIV Medicine* 16 (2008): 62–68.

Chapter 9: Blood Transfusion as a Risk for HIV Infection

Baggaley, Rebecca F., Marie-Claude Boily, Richard G. White, and Michel Alary. "Risk of HIV-1 Transmission for Parenteral Exposure and Blood Transfusion: A Systematic Review and Meta-Analysis." *AIDS* 20 (2006): 805–812.

Constantine, Niel T. "HIV Antibody Testing." In *The AIDS Knowledge Base*, 3rd ed., ed. P. T. Cohen, Merle A. Sande, and Paul A. Volberding, pp. 105–112. Philadelphia: Lippincott, Williams and Wilkins, 1999.

Pilcher, Christopher D., Susan A. Fiscus, Trang Q. Nguyen, Evelyn Foust, Leslie Wolf, Del Williams, Rhonda Ashby, Judy Owen O'Dowd, J. Todd McPherson, Brandt Stalzer, Lisa Hightow, William C. Miller, Joseph J. Eron, Jr., Myron S. Cohen, and Peter A. Leone. "Detection of Acute Infections during HIV Testing in North Carolina." *New England Journal of Medicine* 352 (2005): 1873–1883.

Zou, Shimian, Roger Y. Dodd, Susan L. Stramer, and D. Michael Strong, for the Tissue Safety Study Group. "Probability of Viremia with HBV, HCV, HIV, and HTLV among Tissue Donors in the United States." *New England Journal of Medicine* 351 (2004): 751–759.

Chapter 10: Male Circumcision to Prevent HIV Infection

Gostin, Lawrence O., and Catherine A. Hankins. "Male Circumcision as an HIV Prevention Strategy in Sub-Saharan Africa." *Journal of the American Medical Association* 21 (2008): 2539–2541.

Katz, Ingrid T., and Alexi A. Wright. "Circumcision: A Surgical Strategy for HIV Prevention in Africa." *New England Journal of Medicine* 359 (2008): 2412–2415.

Mandavilli, Apoorva. "Male Circumcision: A New Defense against HIV." *Discover* 29 (2008): 35.

Weiss, Helen A., Daniel Halperin, Robert C. Bailey, Richard J. Hayes, George Schmid, and Catherine A. Hankins. "Male Circumcision for HIV Prevention: From Evidence to Action?" *AIDS* 22 (2008): 567–574.

Chapter 11: Development of an HIV Vaccine

Barouch, Dan H. "Challenges in the Development of an HIV-1 Vaccine." *Nature* 455 (2008): 613–619.

Johnston, Margaret I., and Anthony S. Fauci. "An HIV Vaccine: Challenges and Prospects." *New England Journal of Medicine* 359 (2008): 888–890.

Nkolola, Joseph P., and Max Essex. "Progress towards an HIV-1 Subtype C Vaccine." *Vaccine* 24 (2006): 391–401.

Walker, Bruce D., and Dennis R. Burton. "Toward an AIDS Vaccine." *Science* 320 (2008): 760–764.

Watkins, David I. "Twenty-five Years Later: The Vaccine Search Goes On." *Scientific American* 299 (November 2008): 69–74.

Chapter 12: Evil Spirits and HIV as the Cause of AIDS

Ashforth, Adam. "An Epidemic of Witchcraft? The Implications of AIDS for the Post-Apartheid State." *African Studies* 61 (2002): 121–143.

Dow, Unity. *Far and Beyon'*, 2nd ed. San Francisco: Aunt Lute Books, 2002.

Legare, Cristine H., and Susan A. Gelman. "Bewitchment, Biology, or Both: The Co-Existence of Natural and Supernatural Explanatory Frameworks across Development." *Cognitive Sciences* 32 (2008): 607–642.

Thomas, Felicity. "Indigenous Narratives of HIV/AIDS: Morality and Blame in a Time of Change." *Medical Anthropology* 27 (2008): 227–256.

Chapter 13: Fear and Stigma

Bos, Arjan E. R., Herman P. Schaalma, and John B. Pryor. "Reducing AIDS-Related Stigma in Developing Countries: The Importance of Theory- and Evidence-Based Interventions." *Psychology, Health and Medicine* 13 (2008): 450–460.

Ehiri, John E., Ebere C. Anyanwu, Emusu Donath, Ijeoma Kanu, and Pauline E. Jolly. "AIDS-Related Stigma in Sub-Saharan Africa: Its Contexts and Potential Intervention Strategies." *AIDS and Public Policy Journal* 20 (2005): 25–39.

Holzemer, William L., Leana R. Uys, Maureen L. Chirwa, Minrie Greeff, Lucia N. Makoae, Thecla W. Kohi, Priscilla S. Dlamini, Anita L. Stewart, Joseph Mullan, Ren D. Phetlhu, Dean Wantland, and Kevin Durrheim. "Validation of the HIV/AIDS Stigma Instrument—PLWA (HASI-P)." *AIDS Care* 19 (2007): 1002–1012.

Mahajan, Anish P., Jennifer N. Sayles, Vishal A. Patel, Robert H. Remien, Sharif R. Sawires, Daniel J. Ortiz, Greg Szekeres, and Thomas J. Coates. "Stigma in the HIV/AIDS Epidemic: A Review of the Literature and Recommendations for the Way Forward." *AIDS* 22, Suppl. 2 (2008): S67–S79.

Sweat, Michael, Kevin O'Reilly, Caitlin Kennedy, and Amy Medley. "Psychosocial Support for HIV-Infected Populations in Developing Countries: A Key Yet Understudied Component of Positive Prevention." *AIDS* 21 (2007): 1070–1071.

Chapter 14: Issues of Adolescents and Women

Chersich, Matthew F., and Helen V. Rees. "Vulnerability of Women in Southern Africa to Infection with HIV: Biological Determinants and Priority Health Sector Interventions." *AIDS* 22, Suppl. 4 (2008): S27–S40.

Leclerc-Madlala, Suzanne. "Age-Disparate and Intergenerational Sex in Southern Africa: The Dynamics of Hypervulnerability." *AIDS* 22, Suppl. 4 (2008): S17–S25.

Quinn, Thomas C., and Julie Overbaugh. "HIV/AIDS in Women: An Expanding Epidemic." *Science* 308 (2005): 1582–1583.

Van Damme, Lut, Roshini Govinden, Florence M. Mirembe, Fernand Guédou, Suniti Solomon, Marissa L. Becker, B. S. Pradeep, A. K. Krishnan, Michel Alary, Bina Pande, Gita Ramjee, Jennifer Deese, Tania Crucitti, and Doug Taylor, for the CS Study Group. "Lack of Effectiveness of Cellulose Sulfate Gel for the Prevention of Vaginal HIV Transmission." *New England Journal of Medicine* 359 (2008): 463–472.

Van de Wijgert, Janneke H. H. M., and Robin J. Shattock. "Vaginal Microbicides: Moving Ahead after an Unexpected Setback." *AIDS* 21 (2007): 2369–2376.

Chapter 15: Orphans of HIV/AIDS

Cluver, Lucie D., Frances Gardner, and Don Operario. "Effects of Stigma on the Mental Health of Adolescents Orphaned by AIDS." *Journal of Adolescent Health* 42 (2008): 410–417.

Foster, Geoff. "Supporting Community Efforts to Assist Orphans in Africa." *New England Journal of Medicine* 346 (2002): 1907–1910.

Miller, Candace Marie, Sofia Gruskin, S. V. Subramanian, and Jody Heymann. "Emerging Health Disparities in Botswana: Examining the Situation of Orphans during the AIDS Epidemic." *Social Science and Medicine* 64 (2007): 2476–2486.

Richter, Linda M., and Chris Desmond. "Targeting AIDS Orphans and Child-Headed Households? A Perspective from National Surveys in South Africa, 1995–2005." *AIDS Care* 20 (2008): 1019–1028.

Chapter 16: A Nation Responds

El-Sadr, Wafaa M., and David Hoos. "The President's Emergency Plan for AIDS Relief: Is the Emergency Over?" *New England Journal of Medicine* 359 (2008): 553–555.

Kanki, Phyllis J., and Richard G. Marlink, eds. *A Line Drawn in the Sand: Responses to the AIDS Treatment Crisis in Africa.* Cambridge, Mass.: Harvard Center for Population and Development Studies, 2009.

Ramiah, Ilavenil, and Michael R. Reich. "Building Effective Public-Private Partnerships: Experiences and Lessons from the African Comprehensive HIV/AIDS Partnership (ACHAP)." *Social Science and Medicine* 63 (2006): 397–408.

Steinbrook, Robert. "The AIDS Epidemic: A Progress Report from Mexico City." *New England Journal of Medicine* 359 (2008): 885–887.

Index